Alexander/Kalender/Linke   Computed Tomography

Computed Tomography

Assessment Criteria
CT System Technology
Clinical Applications

by Joachim Alexander, Willi Kalender
and Gerhard Linke

Siemens Aktiengesellschaft

Deutsche Bibliothek Cataloguing in Publication Data:

Alexander, Joachim:
Computed tomography : assessment criteria,
CT system technology, clinical applications /
by Joachim Alexander, Willi Kalender and
Gerhard Linke. Transl. by John McMinn and George
Savatsky. – Berlin ; München : Siemens, [Abt.
Verl.] ; Chichester : Wiley, 1986.
   Dt. Ausg. u.d.T.: Alexander, Joachim:
   Computertomographie
   ISBN 3-8009-1453-0 Pp.
NE: Kalender, Willi:; Linke, Gerhard:

Library of Congress Cataloging-in-Publication Data:

Alexander, Joachim.
   Computed tomography.
   Translation of: Computertomographie.
   Includes bibliographies and index.
   1. Tomography, Emission. I. Kalender, Willi.
II. Linke, Gerhard. III. Title. [DNLM: 1. Tomography,
X-Ray Computed. WN 160 A376c]
RC78.7.T62A4413 1986   616.07'572   86-980

ISBN 0 471 99842 7 (Wiley)

British Library Cataloguing in Publication Data:

Alexander, Joachim
   Computed tomography : assessment criteria,
   CT system technology, clinical applications.
   1. Tomography – Data processing
   I. Alexander, Joachim II. Kalender, Willi
   III. Linke, Gerhard IV. Computertomographie.
   English
   616.07'572   RC78.7.T6
ISBN 0 471 99842 7

Translated by John McMinn and George Savatsky

ISBN 3-8009-1453-0

Editor and publisher: Siemens Aktiengesellschaft, Berlin and Munich
© 1986 by Siemens Aktiengesellschaft, Berlin and Munich
All rights reserved, in particular the rights to reproduce, distribute, translate or otherwise
revise, as well as the use of figures, even for limited purposes. Reproduction and distribution
by means of electronic systems only by written permission of the publisher.

Printed in the Federal Republic of Germany

Contents

Preface 7

Historical Overview 10

1 Evaluation criteria for CT systems – Interpretation of technical data 13
1.1 Image quality 13
1.2 Spatial resolution 13
1.2.1 Modulation transfer function 13
1.2.2 Influence of the system geometry on resolution 18
1.2.3 Influence of the algorithm on resolution 21
1.2.4 Influence of the matrix on resolution 23
1.2.5 Sensitivity profile, slice thickness and dose profile 26
1.3 Noise and noise structure 32
1.3.1 Pixel noise and area noise 33
1.3.2 Noise structure and appearance of the image 35
1.3.3 Noise structure and object form 35
1.4 Contrast-detail diagram 37
1.4.1 Contrast and contrast level discriminating capability 38
1.4.2 Comparison of contrast-detail diagrams for different CT systems 41
1.5 Homogeneity 41
1.5.1 Homogeneity and quantitative image evaluation 41
1.5.2 Homogeneity and the shaping filter 43
1.5.3 Homogeneity and beam hardening correction 43
1.5.4 Beam hardening correction as a compromise 44
1.5.5 Inhomogeneities caused by objects outside of the scan field 46
1.6 Reproducibility 48
1.7 Temporal resolution 49
Literature 50

2 Technology of computed tomography 51
2.1 System concept 51
2.2 Basic types 51
2.2.1 Translation-rotation systems 52
2.2.2 Fan-beam systems 53
2.2.3 Hybrid systems 53
2.3 Detector arrangement 54
2.3.1 Detector geometry, number of detectors and utilization of dose 54
2.3.2 Permissible focal spot size 56
2.3.3 Collimation for scattered radiation 57
2.3.4 Artifact behavior 58

2.3.5	Computed radiography	58
2.3.6	Scanning characteristics	59
2.4	Detector types	61
2.4.1	Detector construction	61
2.4.2	Detector charateristics	62
2.5	Generation of X-ray beam	64
2.5.1	Beam quality	64
2.5.2	Mode of X-ray tube operation	65
2.6	Data processing	69
2.6.1	Hardware	69
2.6.2	Software	77
	Literature	84
3	**Clinical applications of CT systems**	85
3.1	Aspects of routine applications	85
3.1.1	General requirements for operation of a CT system	85
3.1.2	Patient positioning	86
3.1.3	Selection of scanning parameters and flexibility of the examination procedure	89
3.1.4	Image reconstruction and diagnosis	90
3.1.5	Image documentation and archiving	97
3.2	Special applications	97
3.2.1	Optimizing image quality	98
3.2.2	Quantitative computed tomography	102
3.2.3	Dynamic computed tomography	103
3.2.4	Biopsy and stereotaxis	110
3.2.5	Radiation therapy planning	112
3.3	Medical research	114
3.3.1	Problems and goals of CT	114
3.3.2	Example: Evaluation of CT cardiac images	115
3.3.3	Example: Topogram as a diagnostic aid	118
3.3.4	Example: Chronogram	121
3.3.5	Example: Dual-energy method	124
3.3.6	Conclusions	126
	Literature	128
4	**Cost-effectiveness of CT systems**	129
4.1	Amortization and number of examinations	130
4.2	Uniformity of the technical concept	135
4.3	Add-on capability	139
4.4	Standard of quality	141
	Literature	148
Glossary		149

Preface

Computed tomography has become a widely accepted diagnostic modality capable of providing highly detailed diagnostic information with very little risk to the patient. In 1983, there were nearly 7,000 systems in operation. In the same year, over 1,000 additional units were installed. If we combine these figures with the fact that the introduction of computed tomography only goes back about ten years, it then becomes apparent how rapid developments have been.

The striking success of CT was the result of the desire to diagnose pathological processes of the cerebrum with a minimum of risk to the patient and also of the dramatic improvement in CT capabilities.

With the earliest systems, one scan with reconstruction required several minutes. Objects of about 3 mm and density differences of slightly under 1% were detectable. Today, objects considerably smaller than 1 mm and density differences of about 0.3% can be seen within a few seconds. Also remarkable is the simultaneous improvement of all scan parameters.

A description of a modern CT installation would include the following parameters:

Scan times	1 to 10 sec
Reconstruction times	0 to 30 sec
Scan field	42 to 53 cm
Slice thicknesses	1 to 10 mm
Spatial resolution	0.5 to 1 mm
Low contrast detectability	2 to 4 HU
Exposure frequency	8 to 12 min^{-1}

These figures provide a first impression of the capabilities of computed tomography. However in assessing the importance of these factors, it is important to keep in mind that it is the meaningful interplay between these features and not their individual values which are indicative of CT performance. An important goal of this publication is to provide guidelines for more clearly recognizing the scope and value of such data. In addition, there are other influences on the capabilities of computed tomography that cannot be quantified so easily, such as ease of operation, reliability and flexibility.

Even such a detailed examination does not suffice to completely describe modern computed tomography. Whereas the commonly conducted head and whole-body examinations have become so refined that dramatic new developments are unlikely, further development in the realm of special applications will certainly continue.

In keeping with the desire to present as complete a picture of CT tomography as possible, this book has been divided into the following chapters:

Assessment criteria for CT systems
CT system technology
Clinical applications
Cost-effectiveness

Within the limits of the space available, Chapter 3 also gives examples illustrating the main points of emphasis in medical research.

In large university clinics, it is no longer rare to find two or more CT scanners in operation. In small and moderate-sized hospitals, computed tomography is also being introduced at an increasing pace – clearly indicating that this method of examination has become essential for adequate health care.

The impressive growth of computed tomography began in the area of neuroradiology, where it has now become indispensable and supplanted other methods of examination which entail a greater risk to the patient and are of less diagnostic value. With the advent of whole-body computed tomography in a form suitable for clinical application, the diagnostic advantages of CT and its particularly simple examination procedures could be extended to include the entire body.

Some examples of computed tomography supplanting well known methods of examination are:

Pneumencephalography
Cerebral scintiscanning
Cerebral angiography in the cranial region
Myelography
Lymphangiography
Abdominal aortography of the torso

The wide ranging propagation and still widening areas of application for CT owe much to the performance capabilities of the modern whole-body systems available since the beginning of the 80s. Examination of the entire spinal column was made possible with the introduction of a gantry aperture with a diameter of greater than 50 cm. As a result of the considerable freedom offered in positioning the patient, nearly all slice orientations are possible for head examinations. Improved resolution of detail for object sizes in the millimeter range and adaptation of the dose to the type of examination also increase the diagnostic value.

The CT image permits improved morphological discrimination and thus provides important information on the investigation of inner organs and virtually eliminates the need for costly exploratory surgery. The combination of survey radiograms with transaxial slices serves to provide answers to many orthopedic questions. Even in the field of pediatrics, the extremely short scan times and low patient doses favor the use of computed tomography.

This brief account of CT systems suffices to indicate the range of applications of a whole-body CT scanner. In spite of differences in the structure of individual clinics, hospitals and private practices, the vast range of possibilities for utilizing computed tomography, coupled with the quality and diagnostic value of the resulting images, permit its economical operation.

Munich, March 1986

Siemens Aktiengesellschaft

Historical Overview

Even in the very early years of computed tomography, Siemens was able to make significant contributions toward orienting CT technology to the specific requirements of radiologists and X-ray technicians and to help pave the way for CT's wide acceptance.

Since the papers of Hounsfield and Ambrose in 1972 and 1973, there have been three phases of development in computed tomography.

In the initial phase, many firms rushed into development and clinical testing of prototype scanners. Many manufacturers who had no experience in medical X-ray technology also joined in this very competitive race. In this phase, the primary emphasis was clearly to be seen in the development of head scanners.

The EMI scanner developed by Hounsfield was clinically tested in 1973. Only one year later, Siemens was the first producer of medical systems to clinically test a CT scanner – the SIRETOM. Shortly thereafter, Ledley reported on experiments utilizing this new modality for diagnosis of the torso.

The prototype for clinical testing was made available under the name ACTA. The underlying technical principle for these first CT scanners was the linear scanning of the object under study, followed by rotation of the system and repeated scanning. The CT system, consisting of a stationary anode tube together with a mechanically coupled detector, required a few minutes for each scan.

Of particular interest are the technological innovations and characteristics which the SIRETOM introduced into computed tomography. While the EMI scanner still functioned with a time-consuming iterative reconstruction procedure, the Siemens system was even then already using another means of computation – the convolution method. In keeping with this computational procedure, the scanner was equipped with a computer capable of instantaneous image display following each scan. This marked the introduction of convolution and instantaneous image reconstruction into the still new CT technology.

The simple pushbutton operation of the SIRETOM and the, for that time, unusual image display capability via a television monitor are good examples of how Siemens was able to quickly respond to the practical needs of the medical community.

While CT scanners for cranial examinations were being steadily refined until ready for serial production and, parallel to this, computed tomography was gaining wide acceptance in neuroradiology, from 1976 on a second phase of development in CT began to emerge: systems for the examination of the entire body were now being tested.

During this time, Siemens added the Delta Scan 50, manufactured by Ohio Nuclear, to its range of products. With this system, it was possible to scan a transaxial slice in about one minute. At the same time, Siemens was developing a much faster whole-body CT scanner. In this phase, technical innovations made a testing period necessary, which precluded their immediate clinical testing. During this early phase of whole-body computed tomography, developments were fast and furious. Catchwords such as "second", "third" and "fourth" generation signified the rapid advances from one system type to another. In practice, no single design concept was able to assert itself to the exclusion of others.

By the end of 1976, the Siemens SOMATOM whole-body CT scanner was released for clinical operation. It permitted the measurement of one transaxial slice in an unusually large scan field of 53 cm and in a time span of less than 5 seconds with instantaneous image reconstruction. This system was outfitted with the Opti 150 CT high performance rotating anode X-ray tube and the Pandoros Optimatic CT generator, an improved version of the DC generator type already used for cinematic techniques in angiography. They contributed substantially to the SOMATOM's later success. The most efficient utilization of X-radiation within the fan-shaped beam was found to occur with detectors using semiconductor technology. To facilitate problem-free operation in the clinic, all system operation functions were conveniently located at one console and operation was computer guided. At the same time, the $\pm 20°$ range of angulation for the scanning unit permitted direct coronal and sagittal slices of the head.

The initial phases of computed tomography ended by 1979. By then, this new diagnostic modality had become accepted worldwide and Hounsfield and Ambrose received the Nobel prize. By this time, the rapid developments of the earlier years had slowed considerably. Numerous improvements in the systems of the manufacturers still in the CT market made them very suitable for clinical operation. In place of technically interesting designs not ready for operation in practice, a wide variety of applications and the need for reliability now moved into the foreground. The digital survey scan, dynamic scanning techniques, and special procedures for examination of the inner ear, the heart and the spine were all introduced. Increasingly, universal whole-body scanners replaced the early CT head scanners.

The concept of simultaneously rotating the X-ray tube and the detector array around the patient has proven to be reliable and very suitable for routine operation.

Owing to their long scanning times, translation-rotation systems have practically disappeared from the market. Systems utilizing ring detectors show inefficient utilization of radiation and have not been able to establish themselves on the market. The standards by which the performance of a whole-body CT system is measured today are scan times as short as a few seconds, the shortest possible reconstruction times, and the most efficient utilization of radiation.

1 Evaluation Criteria for CT Systems – Interpretation of Technical Data

1.1 Image Quality

From the physical and technical point of view, image quality is a decisive consideration in assessing a CT scanner. In accordance with this, we will first examine some factors contributing to image quality [1].

The two images in Figure 1.1 illustrate a simple but nevertheless interesting manipulation of images, from which we can judge the problems arising in evaluating image quality.

The two CT images are essentially identical, with the only difference being that a "fine-grained" noise has been superimposed onto the lower image. When viewing this image one has the impression that it is sharper than the image above, even though an objective measurement indicates otherwise.

1.2 Spatial Resolution

1.2.1 Modulation Transfer Function

In assessing image quality, spatial resolution is often seen as the most important factor. Viewed within the total context of computed tomography, however, this property should not be accorded such a high importance. The original goal of computed tomography was to be able to distinguish between image details showing only very minute differences in contrast and not to resolve the finest structures. Even today, we should regard the principal field of application for computed tomography as differentiating between soft tissue structures with little difference in contrast.

Nevertheless, in keeping with the usual approach, a few points pertaining to spatial resolution will first be considered, bearing in mind that this concept is, unfortunately, interpreted in different ways.

The limiting spatial resolution from a bore hole test (Fig. 1.2), as seen in the photograph, is the least helpful value. The result of this test – within the limits of the capability to produce bore hole diameters – is the diameter of the smallest test bores still distiguishable.

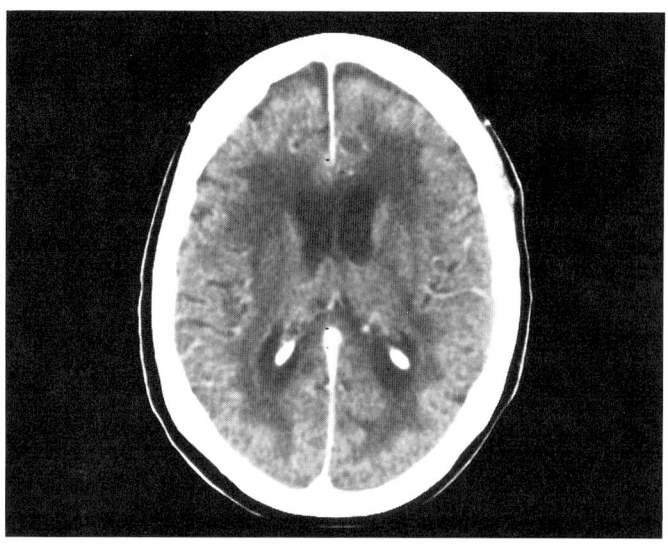

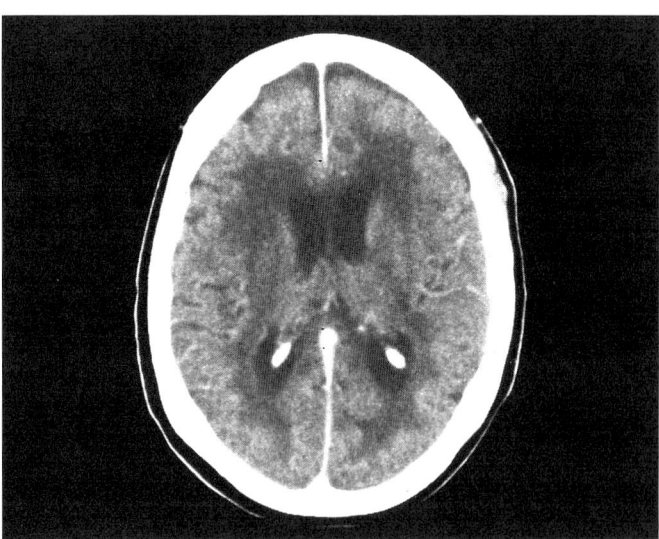

Fig. 1.1
The resolution is identical in both images. The lower appears to be more distinct, due to the presence of superimposed fine-grained noise.

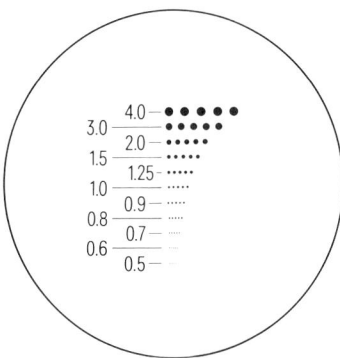

Plexiglas 200 mm ⌀, 15 mm thick
distance between holes equal to diameter

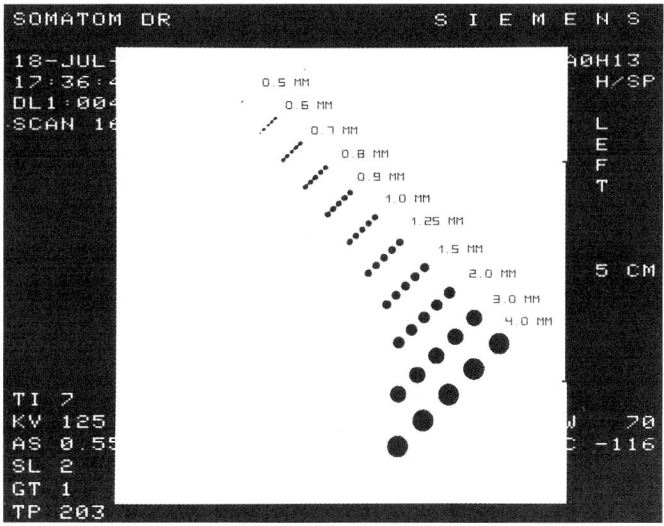

Fig. 1.2
Determination of limiting resolution with the bore hole test

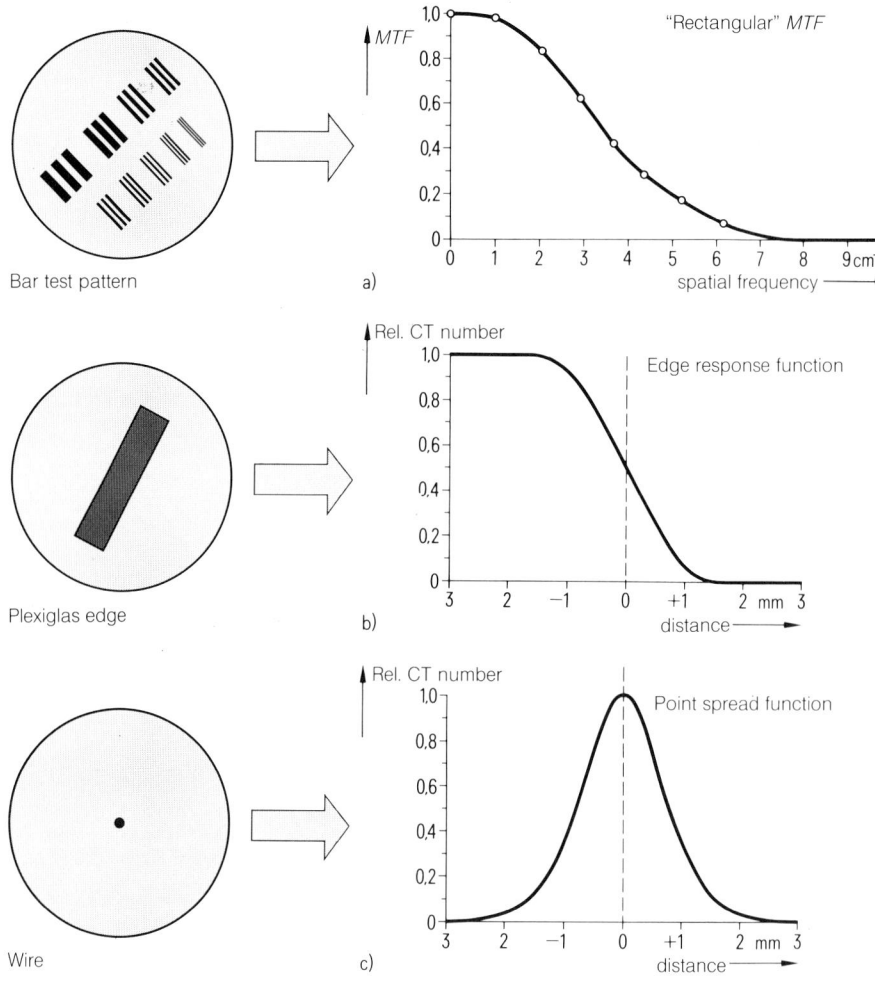

A similar limitation applies to the validity of the limiting frequency for the modulation transfer function (MTF, Fig. 1.3).

A particularly difficult problem already arises in the definition used for limiting frequency. According to manufacturer, the limiting frequency quoted is that for which the MTF has the value 0.05, 0.04 or 0.02. As was true for the bore hole test illustration, the limiting frequency therefore supplies no useful information about the imaging capability for objects larger than those described by the limiting diameter or the limiting frequency.

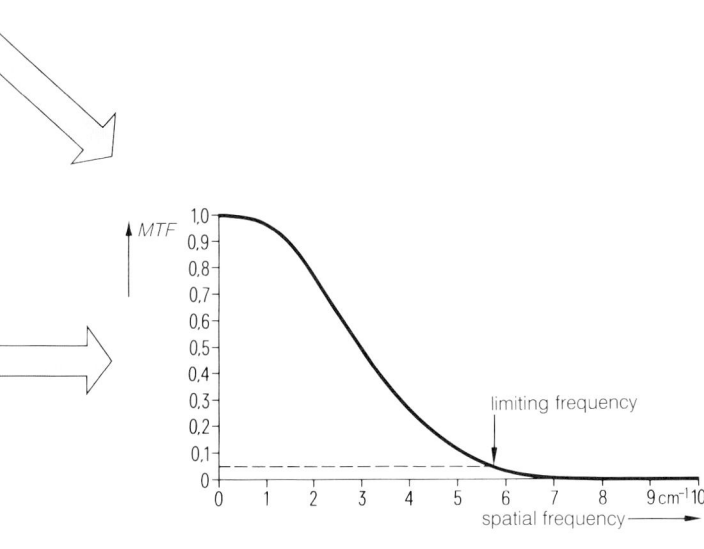

Fig. 1.3
Various methods for determination of the modulation transfer function

The resulting information is valid only for the system MTF in the range of the highest frequency transmitted. For diagnostic purposes, the more important part of the MTF is usually in the range of moderate frequencies (2 to 3 cm^{-1}), and this is then disregarded.

The only useful information in regard to the spatial resolution is then that revealed by the modulation transfer function. Even here, though, it is necessary to observe differences originating in the procedure used for measurement.

Basically, three methods are in use in CT for the determination of the MTF (Fig. 1.3):

▷ "Direct" measurement of the MTF with the aid of a bar test pattern (Fig. 1.3a)

▷ Calculation of the MTF from an edge response function which can be determined with the aid of a plexiglas block in a water phantom (Fig. 1.3b)

▷ Calculation of the MTF from a point spread function developed with the aid of a wire phantom (Fig. 1.3c)

The evaluation of a bar test pattern yields the image contrast or the normalized image contrast as a function of the spatial frequency, but only for a rectangular-shaped modulation function. This does not, however, conform to the definition of the MTF, which assumes a sine wave modulation function.

Since the test objects required to generate such a modulation function can be manufactured only with considerable difficulty, it is in practice necessary to accept the shortcomings of the rectangle test. It is then necessary to calculate a correction to the "rectangular" MTF obtained in order to arrive at the true MTF [2]. Neglecting to perform this correction yields misleading values; because, for a given basic frequency, a rectangular modulation yields a higher contrast level than a sine function. The reason is that, for the same amplitude and frequency, the area under a halfwave rectangular curve is greater than that under a halfwave sine curve. Along with this, for the CT radiograph of a line pair test, there is always a danger that the result is distorted by CT-typical environmental effects and even inadequacies in the beam hardening correction.

The determination of the MTF, for example, from the image of a plexiglas edge entails similar problems: beam hardening errors and environmental effects distort the edge image and therefore also the resulting MTF. Such problems are of no consequence when a point spread function is derived from a scan of a very thin wire (e.g. of 0.1 mm diameter) of material with extremely high attenuation, such as tungsten. The wire can be spanned in air, so that a beam hardening correction becomes unnecessary and, in addition, a practically noisefree scan results. The resulting image is determined only by the system geometry and the image reconstruction algorithm and thus entails only very minute errors in the MTF determination. The basic assumption for the suitability of this method is, however, that the wire can be imaged with the aid of the CT scanner in such a way that the size of the reconstructed pixels remains vanishingly small relative to the expansion of the point spread function. Otherwise, there are simply not enough points measured for the point spread function, so that any further processing of the data becomes uncertain. When the above-mentioned assumption is satisfied, then the MTF should be determined via the scanning of a wire phantom.

1.2.2 Influence of the System Geometry on Resolution

The resolution in the slice plane is determined essentially by the effective width ("beam width") of the individual beam bundles (Fig. 1.4). The effective beam width, B_{total}, is in turn determined by the contribution B_F from the focal spot size, the effective detector width, B_D, and the blurring, B_B, resulting from the motion of the focal spot during the measurement of a value and the ratio of the distances between focal spot, detector and point of measurement. It is assumed that the point of measurement is the center of the field measured. As Fig. 1.4 shows, at this position the motion of the focal spot in a CT scanner (as e.g.

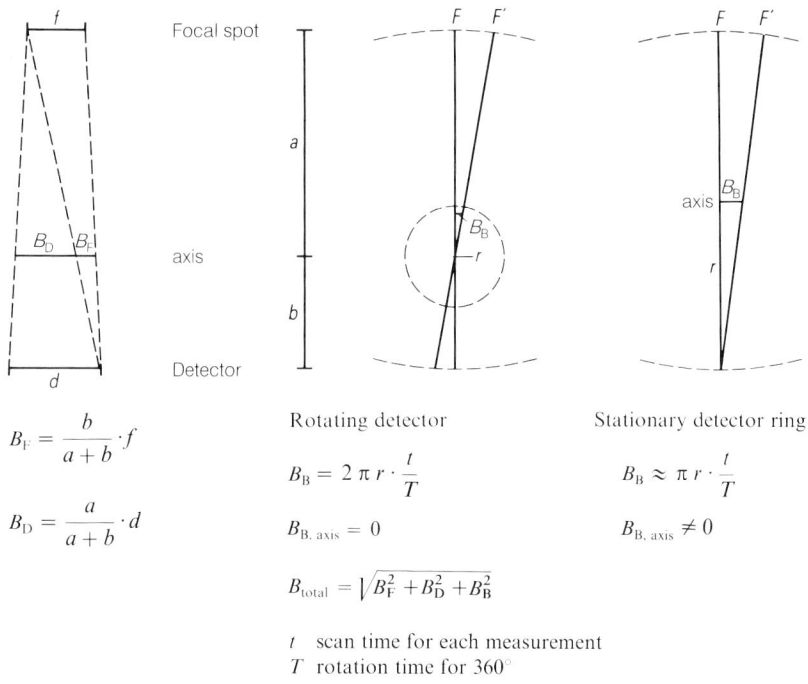

Fig.1.4 Effective width of the beam bundle (beam width)

SOMATOM) for which the detector system moves along with the tube about the object being examined, contributes nothing to the beam width. This no longer applies, however, to a CT scanner with a stationary detector ring (see 2.2).

For any given distance ratios there are two methods of reducing the beam width and thus improving the spatial resolution: using a small (possibly switch-controlled) focal spot and reducing the size of the detector aperture (e.g. by additional collimation). These methods can also be combined. Using a smaller focal spot, however, also entails a reduction of the available X-ray tube output, while reducing the effective detector surface without altering the detector grid gives rise to less efficient utilization of the dose.

In assessing data pertaining to spatial resolution, it is always necessary to consider how these data were obtained with the CT system in question.

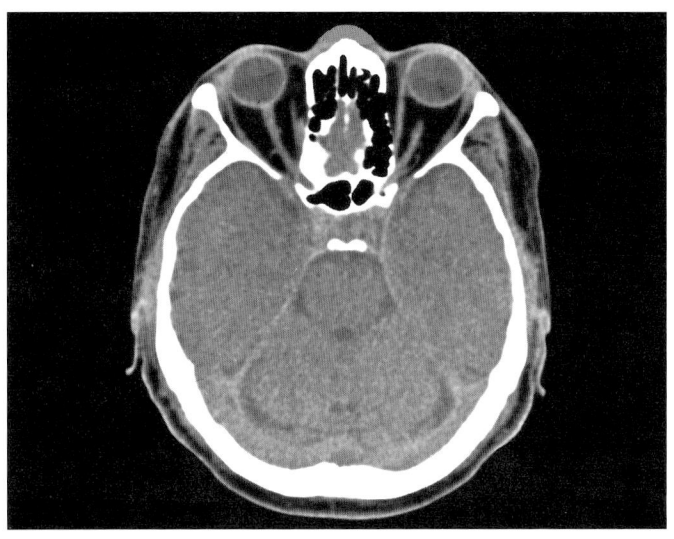

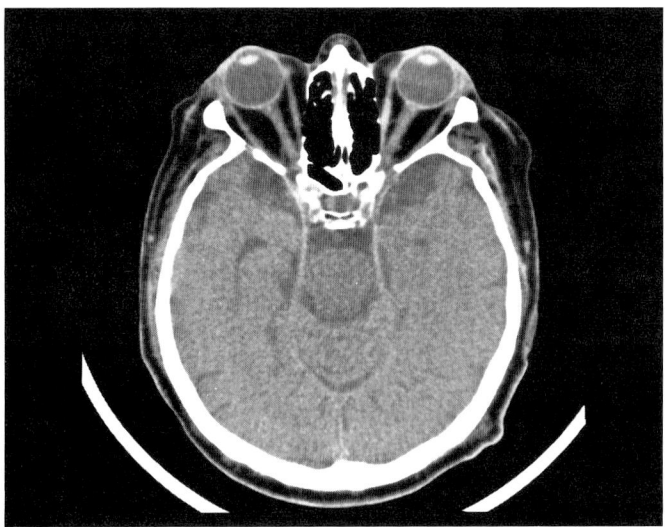

Fig. 1.5a
Effect of a reduction in beam width on the image. Both axial images were obtained with a SOMATOM (above: standard detector array, below: high-resolution detector array).

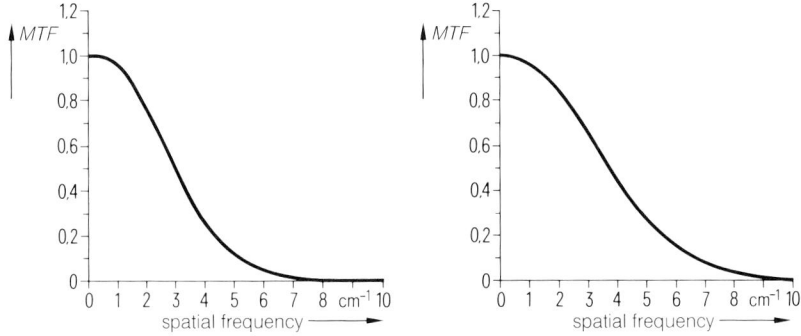

Fig. 1.5b
Effect of a reduction in beam width on the *MTF*.
Left: standard detector array, right: high-resolution detector array.

Figure 1.5 illustrates the effect of a reduction in beam width. Two head scans having nearly the same slice orientation taken from a SOMATOM with a standard detector (512 elements at angular intervals of 5′) and a SOMATOM with a high-resolution detector (704 elements at angular intervals of 3.6′), respectively, are compared. The conditions for scanning and reconstruction were otherwise identical. Fig. 1.5 shows the corresponding modulation transfer functions, as well.

1.2.3 Influence of the Algorithm on Resolution

After the beam width, the most important factor in determining the resolution in the slice plane is the reconstruction algorithm used.

Most CT systems offer the possibility of varying the spatial resolution in the slice plane for a constant geometry by selecting different algorithms (Fig. 1.6). While as a rule the standard algorithm does not come close to reaching the resolution limit inherent in the beam width, algorithms with edge enhancement improve the resolution almost up to this limit.

The use of an edge-enhancing algorithm does, nevertheless, involve two serious disadvantages: the level of image noise is considerably higher, depending on the degree of edge enhancement, and the CT number values for the individual object details are rendered false, thus limiting the quantitative density evaluation of the CT image. With images showing the morphology of high-contrast object structures (e.g. images of the inner ear), though, these limitations are of no importance. Consequently, edge-enhancing algorithms can be used here.

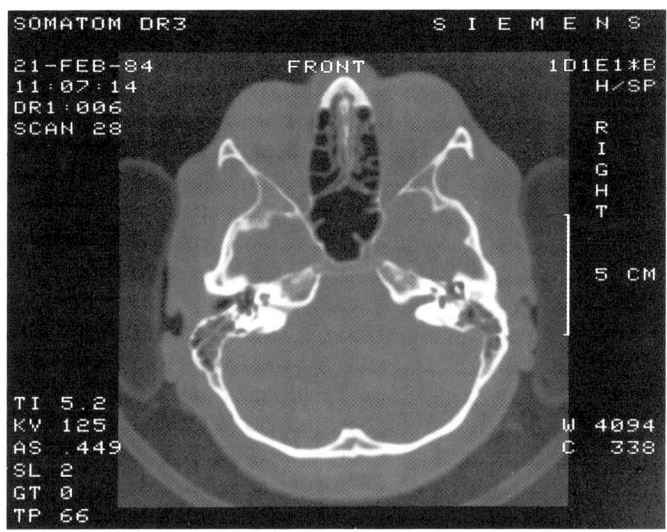

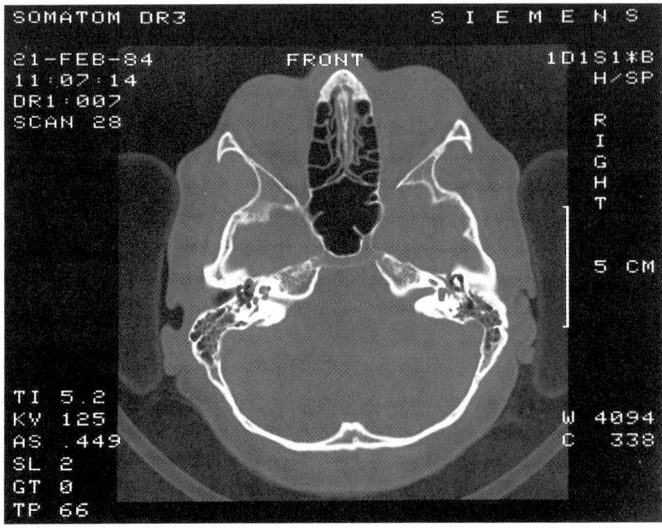

Fig. 1.6a
Influence of the image reconstruction algorithm on resolution. Both images were reconstructed from the same set of data, the upper using the standard algorithm and the lower using a high-resolution algorithm.

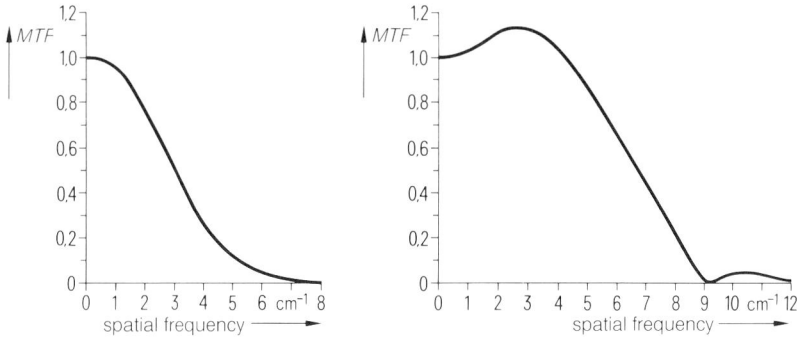

Fig. 1.6b
Influence of the image reconstruction algorithm on the *MTF*.
Left: standard algorithm, right: high-resolution algorithm.

As a result of the disadvantages depicted above, it is always necessary to consider the type of algorithm used in order to correctly judge the resolution. This means that, in comparing different systems, it is ill advised to compare one algorithm without edge enhancement with another edge-enhancing algorithm.

1.2.4 Influence of the Matrix on Resolution

Due to technical and cost effectiveness considerations, it is not possible to reconstruct an image with an arbitrarily large number of pixels. For the SOMATOM DR, the number of pixels is either 512×512 or 256×256. Figure 1.7 illustrates the difference between these two matrix sizes for a head scan. The same data set has been reconstructed first as a 256×256 image (Fig. 1.7, above) and then again as a 512×512 image (Fig. 1.7, below). In the region of soft tissue structures, no appreciable difference can be observed between the two images. On the other hand, for bone contours, it is readily seen that the 512×512 image is considerably smoother. In other words, the range of spatial frequencies which can be represented using a 256×256 matrix suffices, in this example, for the altogether satisfactory reconstruction of the relatively coarse soft tissue structures, but not for the adequate imaging of the marked differences in contrast seen at the edges of bones. It should be pointed out, however, that these are irrelevant to the diagnosis of soft tissue structures.

The limited number of picture elements will limit the resolution of the CT image, at least when the size of the single object elements corresponding to the pixels is larger then the smallest detail which could be resolved by the tube-detector

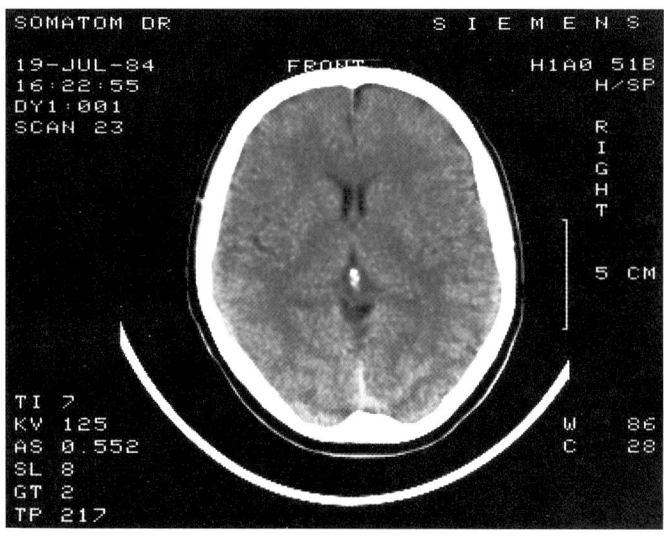

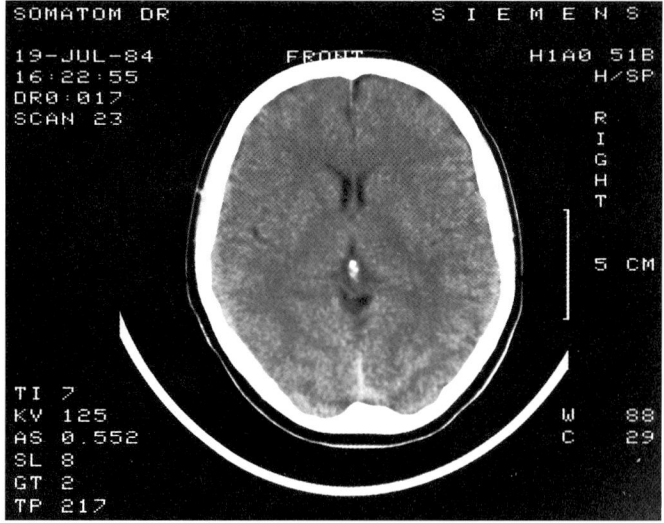

Fig. 1.7
Influence of the matrix on resolution. The images shown were reconstructed from the same data set and the same algorithm, using a 256 x 256 matrix (above) and a 512 x 512 matrix (below).

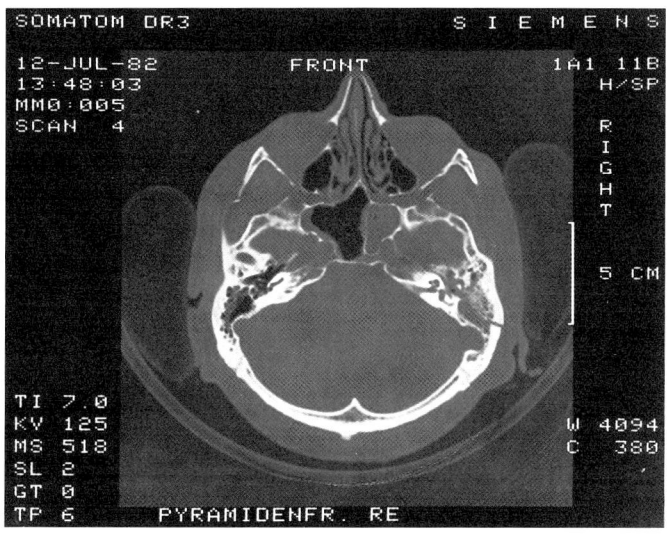
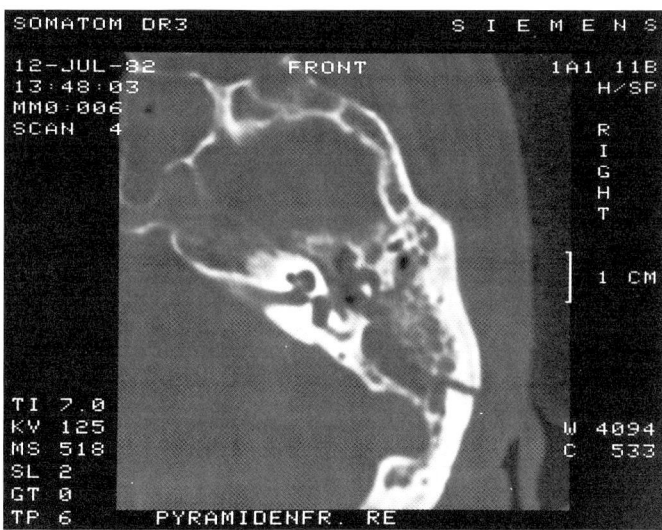

Fig. 1.8
Influence of the image size on resolution. Both images were reconstructed from the same data set using the same algorithm, but with a different zoom factor (above: 2.5, below: 6.0).

arrangement. In order to avoid unduly limiting the resolution capability due to the effect of the matrix, it is necessary to be careful that the diagnostically interesting object range be imaged onto the matrix in such a way that the pixels are small in relation to the object structures of interest or to the smallest detail which the system can resolve. In this regard SOMATOM, through the possible choice of a zoom factor between 1 and 10 and any given center of reconstruction, fulfils the necessary conditions. It is therefore possible to attain the same resolution with a 256×256 matrix as with a 512×512 matrix, as long as the zoom factor is chosen to be twice as large as for the 512×512 matrix, giving the same pixel size in relation to the object. In other words, the 512×512 matrix permits a larger object range than the 256×256 matrix without limiting the resolution.

In clinical practice, it is often necessary to reproduce the entire cross section of the object in a single image for the purpose of orientation and, at the same time, to give the diagnostically important object range with optimum resolution in a second image (Fig. 1.8). It is then particularly advantageous if the CT system offers the possibility for repeated, instantaneous reconstruction from the raw data, as is the case with SOMATOM.

1.2.5 Sensitivity Profile, Slice Thickness and Dose Profile

In discussing the spatial resolution of a CT system, the resolution in the slice plane is often treated completely separately from that perpendicular to the slice plane. In any case, these must satisfy a definite relationship to each other. It would be pointless, for example, to have ten times better resolution in the slice plane than in the plane perpendicular to it. In that case, the form of a single volume element (voxel) corresponding to a pixel (Fig. 1.9) reminds us of a match, i.e. the attenuation properties of the object under investigation are averaged in the slice thickness direction over a disproportionately larger region than in the slice plane. Under these conditions, the high resolution capability in the slice plane can only be meaningfully utilized when the object structures to be imaged run practically parallel to the system axis, which occurs only very infrequently in the human body. Figure 1.10 demonstrates a simple example of the influence of slice thickness on resolution in the slice plane.

High resolution in the slice plane must be balanced by as thin a slice as possible. For technical reasons and also considering the patient dose level, extremely thin layers (below one millimeter) are not possible (see 1.3). As a rule, the slice thickness is defined as the full width at half maximum (FWHM) of the sensitivity profile. This indicates with what level of contrast an extremely thin object in the slice thickness direction is imaged as a function of its position along an axis parallel to the system axis.

The same slice thickness can thus be based on substantially different forms of the sensitivity profile (Fig. 1.11). Since the form of the sensitivity profile determines some of the important system characteristics, it is necessary to know the profile along with the slice thickness in order to assess the image quality of a CT system. The steeper the flanks of the sensitivity profile are, the lower is the contribution of neighboring slices to the slice image in question and the less pronounced is the occurrence of partial-volume artifacts resulting from object details at the edge of the slice which have only been partly detected.

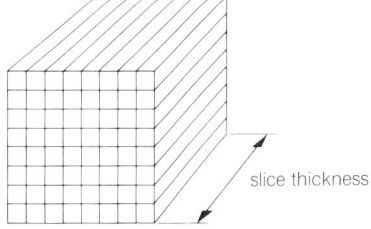

Fig. 1.9
Match-shaped volume element (voxel) for an imbalance between slice plane resolution and slice thickness

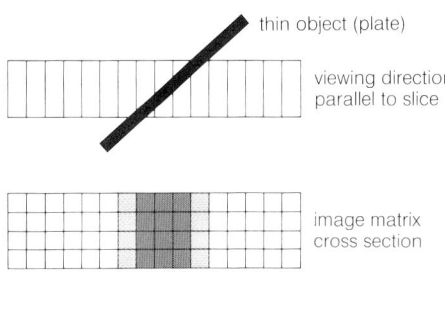

Fig. 1.10
Influence of slice thickness on resolution for object details not aligned parallel to axis

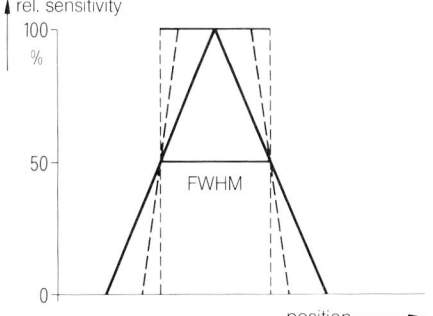

Fig. 1.11
Identical slice thickness for different sensitivity profiles (FWHM: full width half maximum)

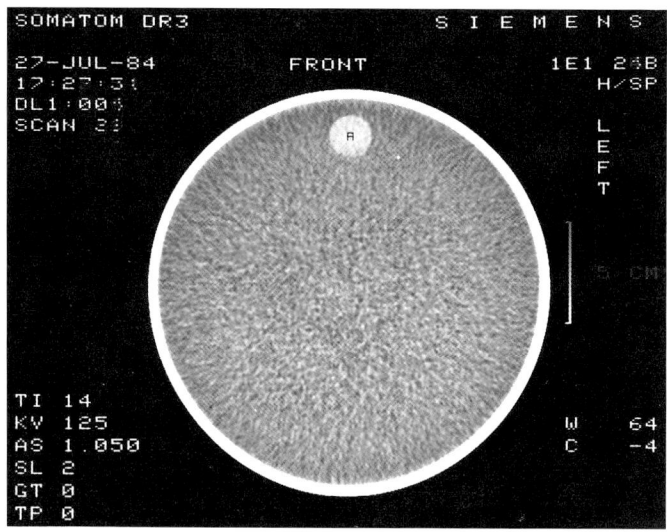

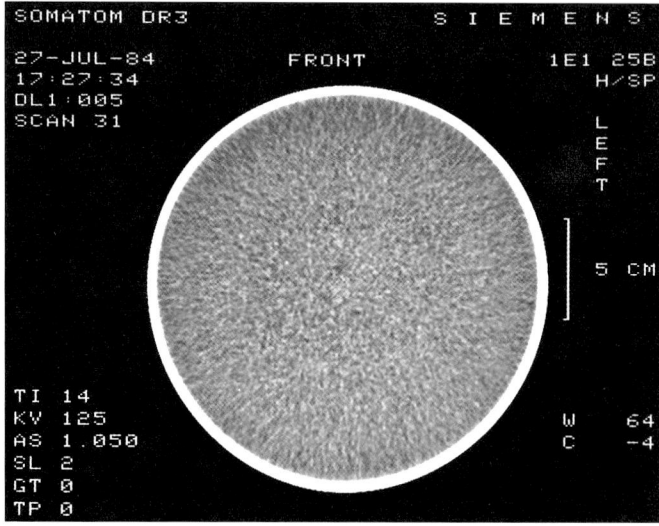

Fig. 1.12a
Contributions from adjacent slices for a strongly trapezoidal (above) and a nearly rectangular (below) sesitivity profile

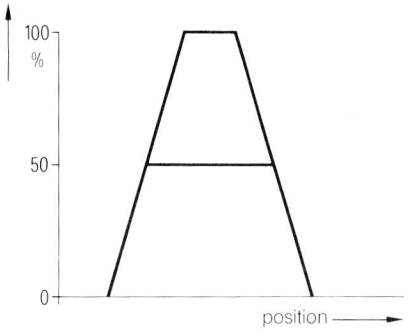 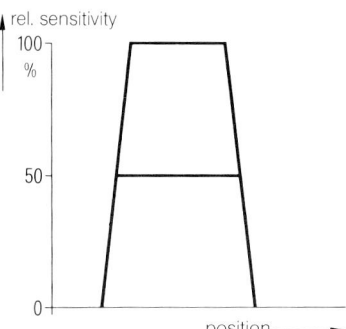

Fig. 1.12 b
Sensitivity profiles for the images in Fig. 1.12 a

Figure 1.12 demonstrates this for two radiographs of a phantom with axial-parallel cylindrical insertions. Both images were obtained using the same phantom position and the same slice thickness, but are derived from different sensitivity profiles. Cylinder A, arranged externally to the slice, with its end surface just tangent to the slice (for a nearly rectangular sensitivity profile) is seen in the image when the sensitivity profile is pronouncedly trapezoidal (Fig. 1.12 a, above), but is no longer present for a nearly rectangular profile (Fig. 1.12 a, below).

It is desirable to make the slice profile as nearly rectangular as possible. Beginning with the assumption that the local sensitivity of the detector is constant in the axial direction, which in practice cannot be satisfied, it would only be possible to achieve a rectangular profile with a focal spot which is infinitesimally small in the axial direction, assuming only a single slice thickness collimator between focal spot and patient, but none between patient and detector (Fig. 1.13). A real focal spot, however, has a finite size and thus produces a penumbra zone at the edge of the collimated radiation beam. This causes a correspondingly flatter rise in the sensitivity profile.

For a given focal spot size, it is only possible to make this rise steeper by placing a collimator before the detector, as shown in Figure 1.13, which either partly or totally blacks out the penumbra region. In addition to positively influencing the sensitivity profile, this collimator also decreases the divergence of the effective

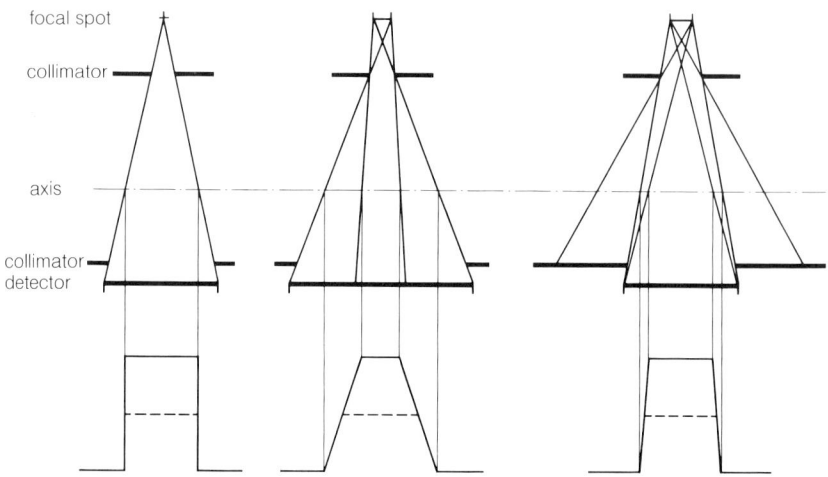

Fig. 1.13
Generation of the most nearly rectangular sensitivity profile by suitable collimation of the radiation beam close to the detector

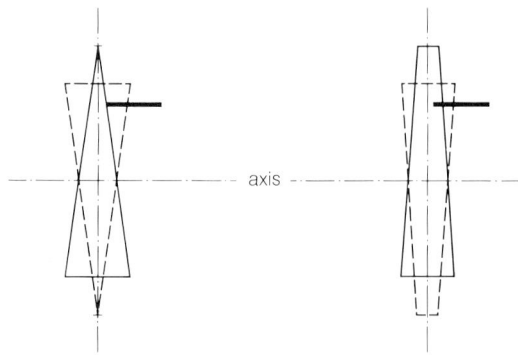

Fig. 1.14
Agreement between oppositely directed projections for different degrees of divergence of the radiation beam in the axial direction

radiation beam between focal spot and detector. This leads to better agreement between beam projections in opposite directions, because outside of the axis even those objects only partly in the slice are evaluated more uniformly (Fig. 1.14).

Owing to the advantages mentioned above, which are particularly noticeable for thin slices, SOMATOM is equipped with such a detector-side collimator for adjustment of the slice thickness. Such a collimator, though, causes radiation which has penetrated the patient in the penumbra zone to go undetected, so that it no longer contributes to the image. The sensitivity profile and the dose profile, i.e. the dose distribution along the system axis, no longer agree (Fig. 1.15). This can be seen, for example, in the increased surface dose in the images for a series of immediately adjacent slices, when compared with the image of a single slice. The factor by which the dose is found to increase is called the pile-up factor.

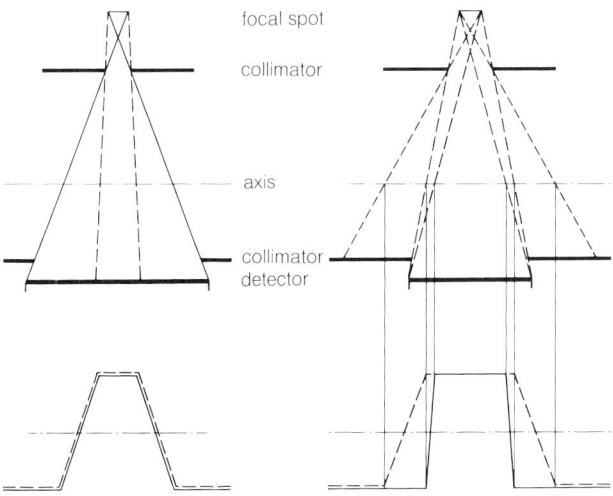

Fig. 1.15
Sensitivity profile and dose profile without (left) and with (right) beam collimation between object and detector

Owing to their design (without detector-side slice collimation), some CT systems show very good agreement between the sensitivity profile and the dose profile. However, even in these systems the pile-up factor significantly exceeds the ideal value of 1, because of the contribution due to scattered radiation. The enhancement of the pile-up factor through the use of detector-side slice collimation is thus not as great as might first be expected on the basis of idealized considerations.

This is particularly true when, as for SOMATOM, a well considered compromise is chosen, and the penumbra zone is not blackened out entirely. The FWHMs of the dose profile and the sensitivity profile then differ only slightly. In a comparison of CT scanners, the dose pile-up factor alone tells us very little. It describes only a part of the total patient dose efficiency of a CT system, but still ignores e.g. the following consideration: due to its high power, a relatively large focal spot, producing a broad penumbra zone and resulting in a correspondingly large pile-up factor when this zone is blackened out, allows more effective filtration of the beam for a given signal strength. This means that the patient dose can be reduced at least as much as the pile-up factor increases when a large focal spot is used in place of a small focal spot with a minimum of filtration, provided that the filter and focal spot are correctly dimensioned.

The dose pile-up factor must always be viewed in relation to the absolute dose figures and the resolution and noise level values attained. Much more complete information on the dose generated by a CT system is given by the CT dose index (CTDI). The CT dose index is the quotient of the dose line integral – the integral of the local dose over the entire dose profile in the axial direction – and the slice thickness. Citing the CTDI excludes any possible confusion (such as due to different numbers of slices) inherent in the pile-up factor.

1.3 Noise and Noise Structure

Next to spatial resolution, pixel noise is the image quality parameter most frequently investigated and discussed. There are many variables and processes leading to and affecting pixel noise, of which the most important are quantum noise resulting from the X-radiation detected, noise originating in electronic components and the reconstruction algorithm.

The level of quantum noise in the radiation detected depends upon the level generated at the X-ray tube, the filtration used, the slice thickness selected, the beam attenuation in the object and the absorption capacity of the detector.

1.3.1 Pixel Noise and Area Noise

When speaking of noise, it is often only the pixel noise which is meant. Quantitatively, this is the standard deviation of the CT values in the image of a homogeneous phantom within a test area of given size and form. Due to the simplicity of its measurement, this is the most widely used measure of noise, but by itself it is not suitable for comparing CT scanners. It should always be examined in conjunction with the spatial resolution in the slice plane, the slice thickness, the dose, and the attenuation characteristics (thickness and material) of the test object.

Figure 1.16 depicts the influence of the algorithm employed on the noise. The two images were reconstructed from the same set of data by means of a standard algorithm and a high-resolution algorithm (see 1.2.3). The high-resolution algorithm also entails a higher noise level.

With a carefully dimensioned CT scanner, apart from extreme operating conditions the contribution of electronic noise to the pixel noise is negligible in comparison with the contribution arising from quantum noise. It then follows that the pixel noise level is inversely proportional to the square root of the dose absorbed (for constant X-ray tube voltage and filtration) and inversely proportional to the square root of the slice thickness. SOMATOM fulfils these conditions over a very wide range. If deviations from these relations are found in testing the scanner (Fig. 1.17), then there are other sources of noise in addition to quantum noise for the scanner tested and the radiographic conditions chosen.

Pixel noise is essentially a variable which without much effort permits controlling how satisfactorily a single scanner is operating or comparing several scanners of the same model. For this purpose it is only necessary to compare the current noise level with the results of earlier measurements. If it is desired to describe with what probability an object of given size and having a given contrast level can be detected with different types of scanners, it is necessary to determine at least the area noise level. This is the standard deviation of the average CT values over small test areas, corresponding to the object of interest, in the image of a homogeneous phantom. This is the only way to take into account that there is an interplay of pixel noise between the individual pixels. This correlation of noise level values derives from the contribution of each value measured (with different weighting of the single values) to each pixel. It is a consequence of the reconstruction process. The immediate result of this is the visible noise structure, present in every CT image.

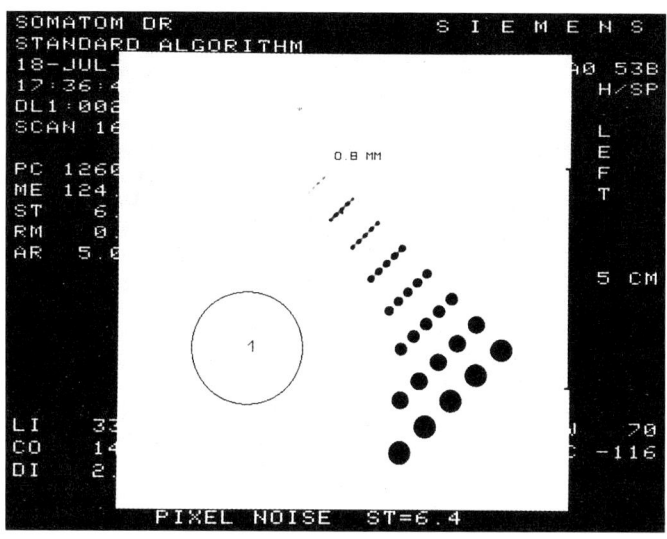
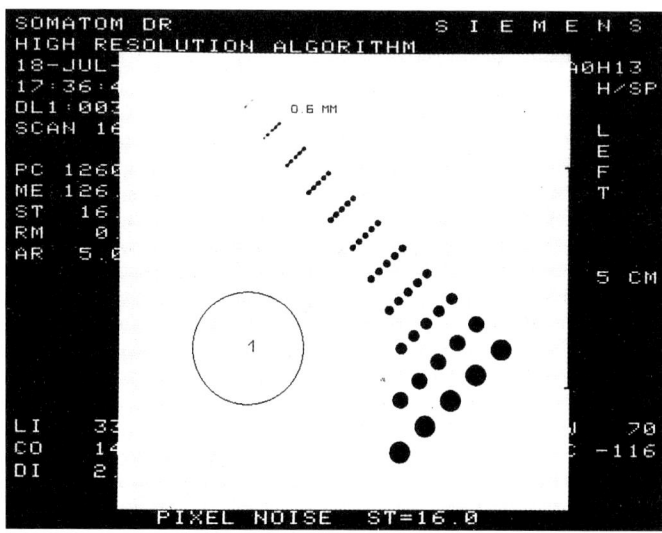

Fig. 1.16
Noise and resolution for different algorithms. The two scans were constructed from the same set of data. The lower-resolution algorithm (above) gives rise to a lower noise level than the higher-resolution algorithm (below).

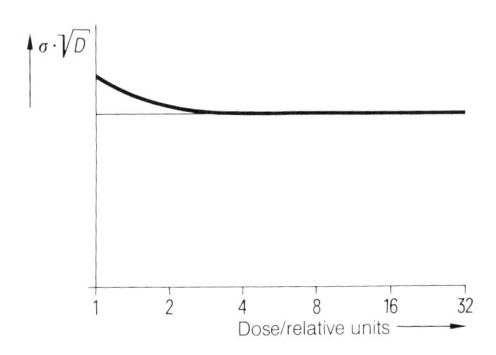

Fig. 1.17
Product of noise level and square root of dose as a function of dose with other sources of noise present in addition to quantum noise. Without such additional sources of noise, this product would be constant.

1.3.2 Noise Structure and Appearance of the Image

The noise structure evident in the image has a considerable effect on the degree of sharpness which the viewer perceives in a CT image. Coarse-grained noise gives the immediate impression of a blurred image, even if the spatial resolution capability of the scanner is good. Fine-grained noise, on the other hand, gives a false impression of sharpness, even if the quality of image resolution is inferior. Figure 1.1 shows the results of a pertinent experiment. A strictly visual appraisal would be altogether disastrous for the conditions simulated; it is necessary to formulate an objective criterion for assessing image sharpness.

1.3.3 Noise Structure and Object Form

The cross section of the human body can be described as approximately elliptical. As a result of this form, there is a noise structure typical of CT images. Figure 1.18, which shows a CT radiograph from a cylindrical water phantom, illustrates this. Indistinct, radially oriented structures can be seen clearly at the edge of the object under study. This noise pattern arises from the fact that the object becomes gradually thinner toward the edge, with the result that the radiation is attenuated more strongly along a diameter then along a secant. Consequently, the signal measured contains widely different levels of quantum noise in directions perpendicular to each other, in turn giving rise to obvious structures in the images viewed.

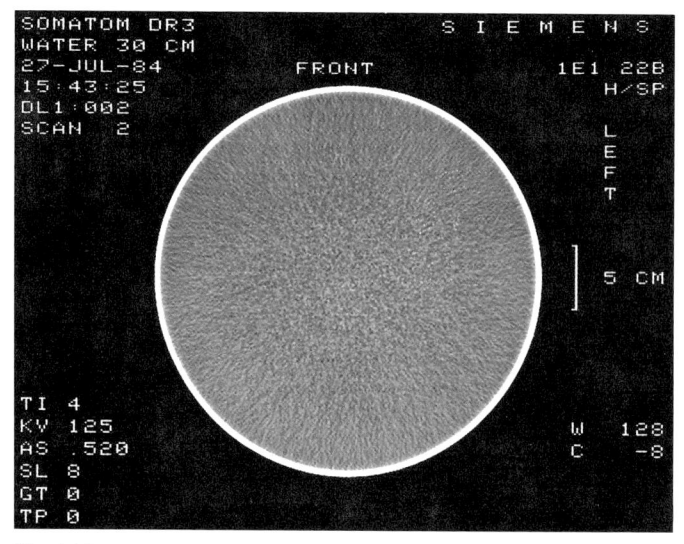

Fig. 1.18
Radially oriented noise structures resulting from different noise levels of the central and peripheral parts of the radiation beam penetrating the object

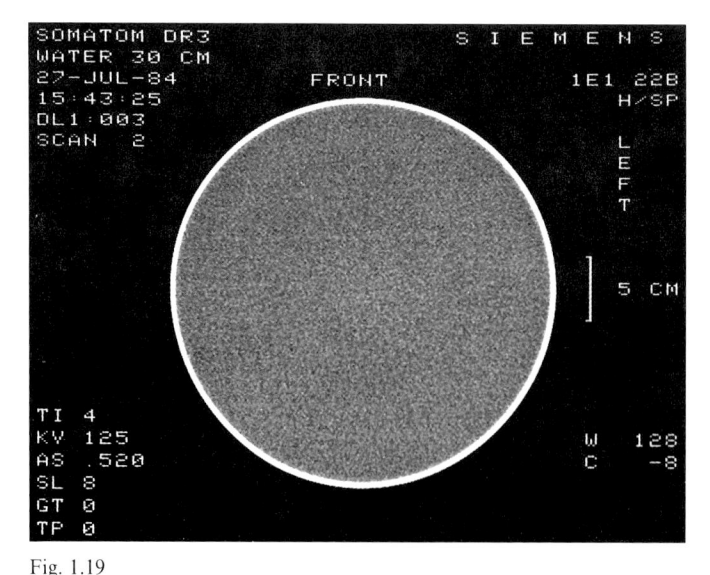

Fig. 1.19
Suppression of the radial noise structures through insertion of a filter tailored to the object examined. Here, the result of a corresponding computer simulation with noise enhancement in the peripheral signals prior to reconstruction.

Through the use of a shaped filter adapted to the body cross section, it is possible to attenuate all parts of the radiation beam almost uniformly, thus suppressing such noise structures. The results of an experiment simulating these results are shown in Figure 1.19. For SOMATOM, such a shaping filter was intentionally not included: the advantages for image quality (less noise structures) are counterbalanced by considerable disadvantages, particularly inadequate homogeneity of the image in the event that the shaping filter cannot be fitted at all or only inadequately to the object (see 1.5.2).

1.4 Contrast-Detail Diagramn

The modulation transfer function describes only the spatial resolution capability, while area noise allows us to assess the expected low contrast detectability. The contrast-detail diagram [3] yields information on the resolution capability relative to the object size and at the same time to the variations in density of the object details (see Fig. 1.20). All object details for which the coordinates intersect above

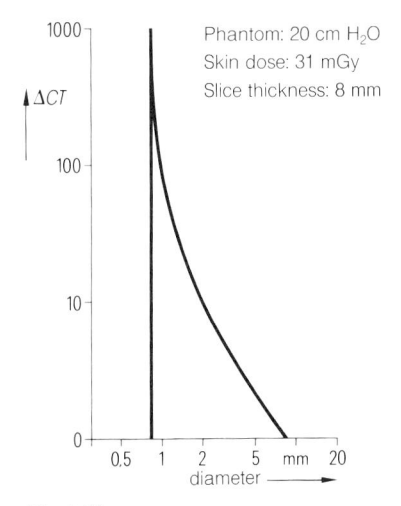

Fig. 1.20
Typical contrast-detail diagram. Using the scanning parameters given next to the curve, the CT system can only image those details for which the contrast and diameter coordinates intersect above the indicated boundary line.

the curve indicated in this diagram can be imaged, and all other details cannot. Owing to this wide ranging statement, the contrast-detail diagram is of particular importance in assessing the image quality of a CT scanner and must therefore be determined with utmost care and objectivity.

1.4.1 Contrast and Contrast Level Discriminating Capability

In the classical method for determining a contrast-detail diagram, a cylindrical phantom with groups of bore holes (Fig. 1.21) is used. In principle, this is similar to the bore hole test used for determining the limiting spatial resolution, except that now the contrast of the bore holes in relation to the surroundings can be varied by filling the phantom with liquids of different attenuation properties.

When a phantom of this type is used in order to compare the contrast-detail diagrams for different CT systems, it is usually assumed that, for the same filling, the phantom yields the same contrast level for all CT systems. That this assumption is untenable can be seen from Figure 1.22. The two scans were performed using the same phantom at two different X-ray tube voltages for the same scanner. It is seen that the contrast level is strongly dependent upon the beam quality (see 2.5.1). The importance of this statement can be appreciated when it is pointed out that different CT systems utilize differing beam qualities.

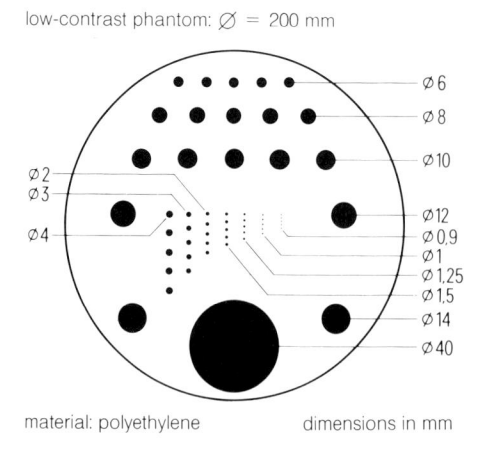

Fig. 1.21
Phantom for determination of the contrast-detail diagram

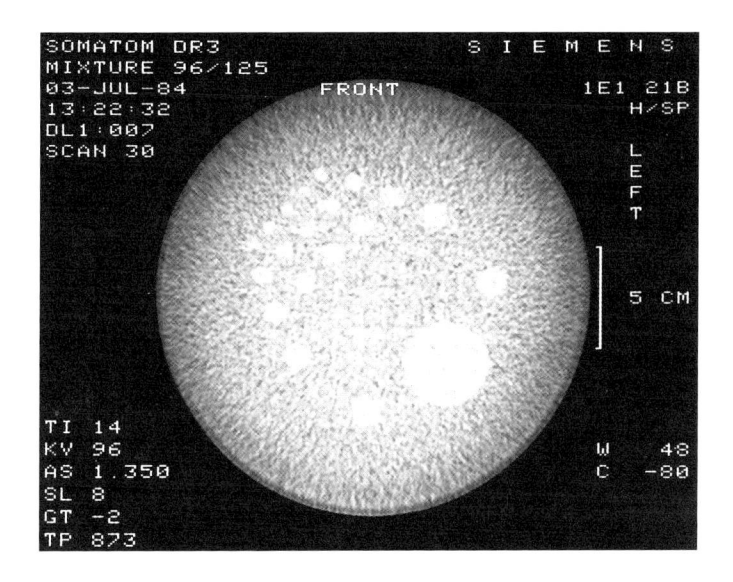

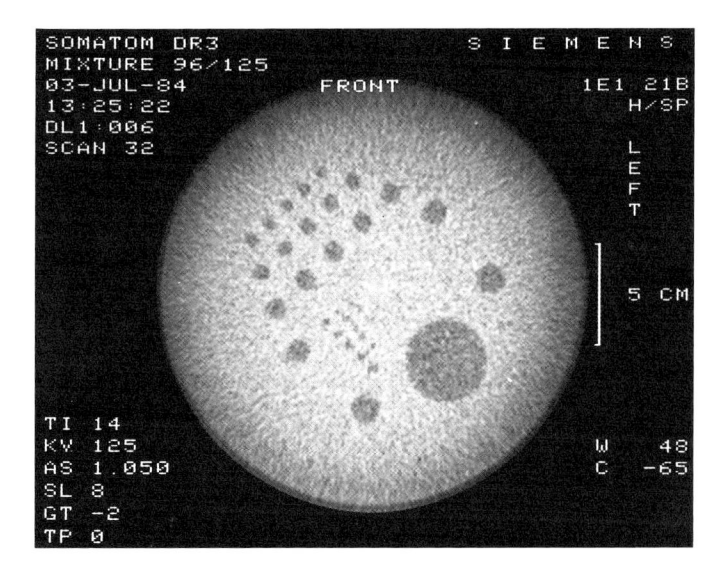

Fig. 1.22
Dependence of the contrast level for the phantom filling on beam quality. The two scans were made using the same phantom with the same filling, for two different X-ray tube voltages (above: 96 kV, below: 125 kV).

The contrast level actually attained with the filling must therefore always be carefully determined with sufficiently large test areas. The diameter of the smallest recognizable test bore holes corresponding to this contrast level value are then entered in the contrast-detail diagram.

Only in this way is it possible to distinguish clearly between the contrast level attained for the phantom in the individual CT scanners and the applicable contrast discrimination capability.

The risk of not adequately differentiating between contrast level and contrast discrimination capability and, at the same time, the uncertainty of the classical method for determination of the contrast-detail diagram, caused by the subjective nature of visual observations, can be avoided by using a new type of method, which we proposed some time ago [4]. In this method, the contrast-detail diagram is determined from the modulation transfer function and the noise level in the image from a homogeneous water phantom. Assuming noisefree imaging, for a given level of object contrast and an arrangement of test bodies corresponding to the bore hole phantom, the level of image contrast can be calculated from the MTF as a function of the object diameter. The noise level for the contrast of the test bodies relative to their surroundings can be taken from the water phantom scan, as this noise level is equal to that from the difference of the average CT values within neighboring circular areas for different positions in the image of the water phantom. This assumes that the diameter of these circular areas is the same as that of the test objects. The quotient of this noise level and the calculated image contrast level is proportional to the minimum contrast level needed to recognize the test objects. This level is represented in the contrast-detail diagram as a function of the object diameter.

1.4.2 Comparison of Contrast-Detail Diagrams for Different CT Systems

Just as for noise at a given object diameter, the minimum contrast level, ΔCT, required for recognition also depends upon the effective dose seen at the detector. In fact, it is inversely proportional to the square root of the dose. The dose seen at the detector is proportional to the surface dose, D, at the object and the slice thickness, t. If two scanners A and B differ in the skin dose and the slice thickness, the following formula compares their necessary minimum contrast values:

$$\Delta CT_A = \Delta CT_B \cdot \sqrt{\frac{D_B \cdot h_B}{D_A \cdot h_A}}$$

If for a given object diameter the minimum contrast level for scanner A, as read from the contrast-detail diagram, is less than ΔCT_A, then scanner A has the better contrast discrimination capability for this object diameter.

It is considerably more difficult to make such a comparison if the two contrast-detail diagrams are derived using phantoms having different attenuation capacities, resulting from differences in material or thickness. In this case, it is necessary to know the beam quality very well in order to determine the corresponding differences in dose. The rule of thumb that three centimeters of water cause a factor of two change in the signal measured can easily lead to intolerably high errors. Contrast-detail diagrams can only be compared when the dose and the slice thickness are given, using the same method of measurement and, if possible, the same type of phantom (material and size).

1.5 Homogeneity

1.5.1 Homogeneity and Quantitative Image Evaluation

An important characteristic far too often neglected in assessing the image quality of a CT scanner is the homogeneity. This is a measure of the uniformity in the average CT value of a material over the entire image cross section in the image of a homogeneous phantom. The degree of homogeneity contributes to determining whether a tissue region is imaged with the same average CT value at different positions in the cross sectional image of a body. It is therefore a value of particular interest for quantitative diagnoses.

When diagnosing from CT scans, the question of morphology remains the most important. At the same time, the importance of quantitative information based upon a density determination is increasing continuously. SOMATOM takes this tendency into account through particularly good homogeneity characteristics (Fig. 1.23).

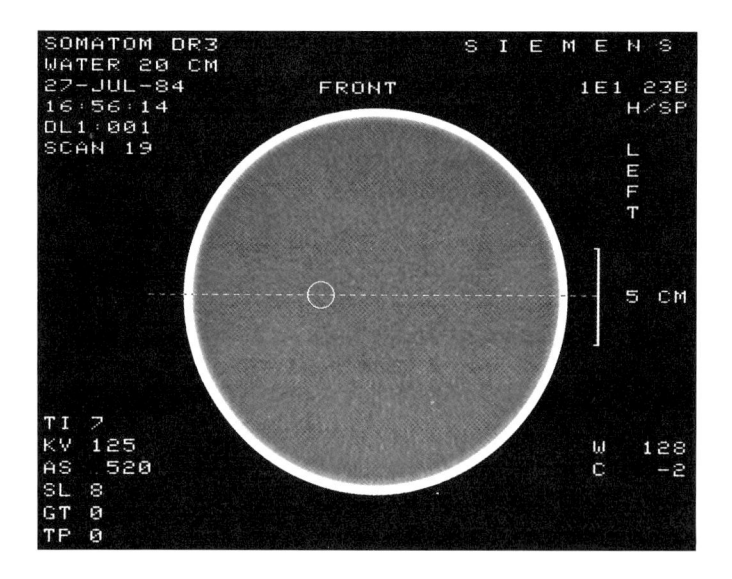

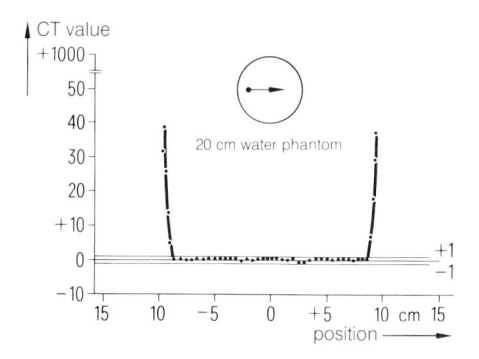

Fig. 1.23
Homogeneity of the SOMATOM DR
The values shown in the diagram are the average CT values within circular areas of about 1 cm² along the line shown in the image of the 20 cm water phantom

1.5.2 Homogeneity and the Shaping Filter

As already mentioned in section 1.3.3, a shaping filter fit to the size of the object to be scanned helps to reduce aesthetically disturbing noise structures and to homogenize the noise. At the same time, such a filter lowers the signal level seen at the detector. For detectors having a limited range of modulation (for example, due to saturation, such as for an inert gas detector: see 2.4), this can be advantageous.

The disadvantage is that the correct use of a shaping filter requires an individual beam hardening correction for each channel measured, because each radiation beam has a different beam quality. This, of course, leads to a substantially more complicated data correction procedure. As a rule, such a procedure must therefore involve compromises in regard to the integrity of the beam hardening correction. For reasons of technology and cost-effectiveness, it is not possible to equip a CT system with a wide variety of shaping filters matching a vast range of different object sizes. In general, there are only two shaping filters supplied with such scanning systems.

Such methods only produce homogeneous images when the size and material of the object under study are well matched to the shaping filter used. If the object deviates in its size or its attenuation characteristics from the standard object or if the object is not centered exactly in the scan field, then marked inhomogeneities can occur in the form of vignetting.

Because of these disadvantages, shaping filters are not used with SOMATOM.

1.5.3 Homogeneity and Beam Hardening Correction

In order to be able to generate the desired high beam intensities with sufficiently small source areas, X-ray tubes are almost always used to generate CT beams. Only a few dedicated systems use different radiation sources (i.e. isotope systems).

X-ray tubes emit a broad spectrum of X-ray quanta having various energies, which are in turn attenuated differently in the object under study. As a result, the effective energy of the radiation spectrum is shifted after passing through the object to increasingly higher values as the object thickness increases. Before reconstructing images from the data measured, it is necessary to correct for this beam hardening effect (Fig. 1.24). Otherwise, the data measured from different directions of projection, in which different object thicknesses are in effect documented, would not fit together.

It can be appreciated at once that an insufficient or incorrect beam hardening correction adversely affects the homogeneity. For this reason, SOMATOM has

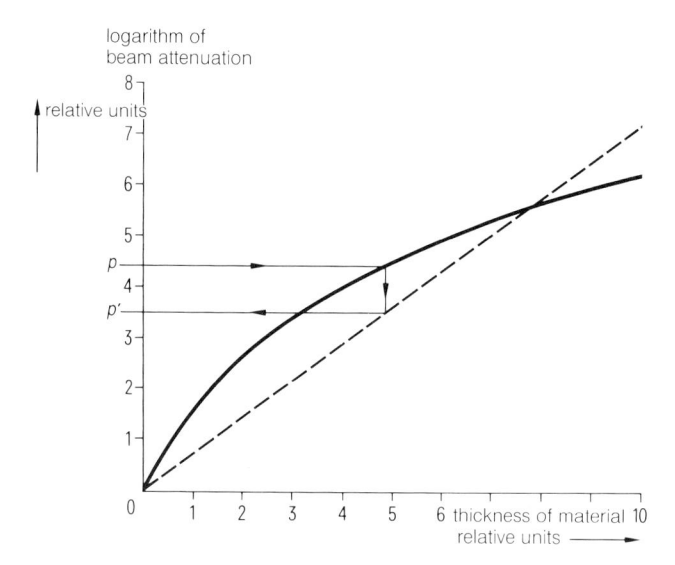

Fig. 1.24
Beam hardening correction
Distortions in values measured caused by changes in the spectrum in passing through the object are corrected so that for a given material the assumed linear relation between object thickness and logarithm of attenuation is reproduced

given special attention to this point. An important factor in preventing beam hardening artifacts is the use of a 0.25 mm or (with the newest SOMATOM models) even 0.4 mm thick copper filter, in addition to the inherent filtration of the X-ray tube by 2.5 mm (aluminum equivalent). This filter already narrows the spectral width considerably, so that the hardening effect is no longer as pronounced. A computer correction to the beam hardening is then possible over a wide range of object thicknesses.

1.5.4 Beam Hardening Correction as a Compromise

In principle, the effectiveness of a beam hardening correction is limited, if we assume an attenuation capacity of the object determined from only one beam spectrum. It is not possible to differentiate between attenuation resulting from a thick layer of a largely non-hardening material, such as plexiglas, or from a thinner layer of more strongly hardening material, such as aluminum. If the composition of the object deviates very much from that assumed in determining the beam hardening correction, the correction will not be effective and it will not be possible to prevent the appearance of artifacts (e.g. between the petrous bones in a head scan: see Fig. 1.25).

Such artifacts can sometimes be corrected later, if the positions of boney layers are known from the reconstructed image. Only the dual-energy method provides a reliable means of suppressing these artifacts, by examining the object with two different beam spectra. For routine examinations, however, such a method is too cumbersome, with the result that the usual beam hardening correction must still be used. As we have already seen, this can only be regarded as a compromise solution.

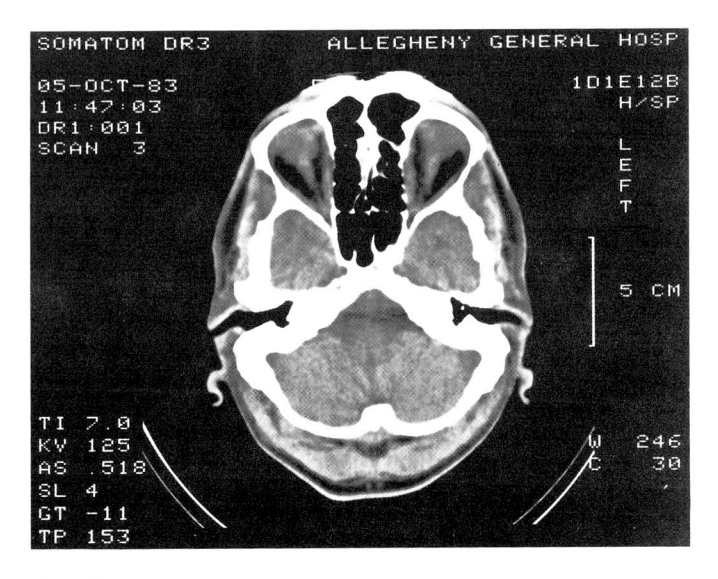

Fig. 1.25
Typical petrous bone artifact
The hardening effects can only be partially corrected, since the object is not sufficiently water equivalent

1.5.5 Inhomogeneities Caused by Objects Outside of the Scan Field

As for the case of no beam hardening correction, discrepancies occur in the values measured between different directions of projection if parts of the object in the slice region project beyond the limits of the scan field (Fig. 1.26). Parts of objects located outside the scan field cause vignetting, which is more pronounced toward the periphery of the scan field and precludes a quantitative determination of density. With the aid of plausible assumptions regarding the object form, it is possible in such cases to apply corrections to the data and thus reduce inhomogeneities. Optimum results, however, require that the object under examination does not extend beyond the limits of the scan field. The simplest way of guaranteeing this is to use a large scan field (for SOMATOM, about 50 cm in diameter). It is then no longer necessary to exercise extreme care in positioning the patient.

For a fan-beam scanner (see 2.2), such as SOMATOM, it is no longer even necessary to determine the entire cross-section in each projection. In principle, it is sufficient to utilize only one half of the scan field, as long as the system rotates through an angle of at least 360°. For the SOMATOM CR, the lowest-priced SOMATOM model, this has been done up to a point. The central scan field, having a diameter of 29 cm, with which in regard to spatial resolution the most difficult objects (head and spine) are studied, is detected in its entirety. The edge zone projecting beyond it is only detected on one side.

As a result, no significant loss in resolution occurs in the peripheral region. The noise level is higher in the peripheral region, but in general the object to be scanned is thinner than in the center of the scan field. Considering this, such an arrangement of detectors gives rise to a certain homogenization of noise, much as with a shaped filter. The special detector configuration for the SOMATOM CR does not give inhomogeneities in the CT values, because here as well the entire scan field is measured.

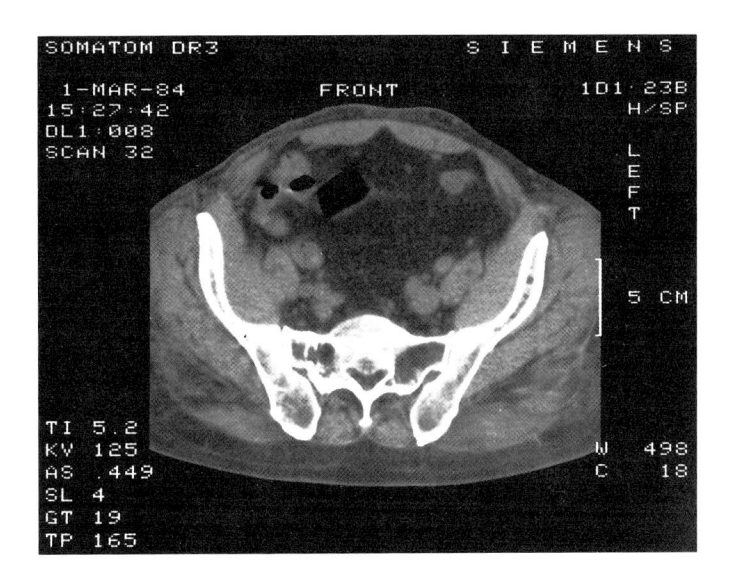

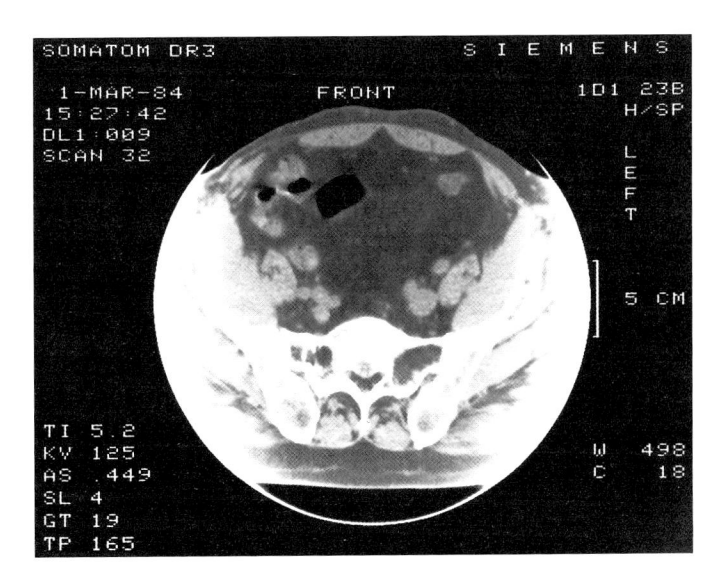

Fig. 1.26
Vignetting due to object parts outside of the scan field. From the data set yielding the image above, a second image considering only the middle 256 channels was reconstructed.

1.6 Reproducibility

It is extremely important for the user to be able to consistently obtain the same image – within well-defined tolerances – from the same object, using the same scanning parameters. Follow-up studies using CT will only be meaningful when this requirement has first been satisfied.

In order to guarantee good image reproducibility, it is necessary to maintain a constant level of beam quality and dose and also to prevent the occurrence of system-generated artifacts.

For a given anode material and filtration, the beam quality depends only upon the voltage of the X-ray tube and the surface characteristics of the anode. A rough anode surface, such as caused by local overheating during operation, causes excessive inherent filtration. A suitable choice of generator allows maintaining a constant voltage level for the X-ray tube. A careful consideration of the loading capacity for the anode is necessary in determining the scanning parameters, so that roughening of the anode surface is reduced to a minimum.

For SOMATOM, either the secondarily regulated (i.e., from the high-voltage side) and switched PANDOROS CT or the regulated medium-frequency MICROMATIC generator is used, depending upon the scanner type. Both yield sufficient reproducibility of the X-ray tube voltage.

For the scanning parameters needed in computed tomography, it is not possible to prevent roughening of the anode altogether. With SOMATOM, operating the anode below maximum loading capacity (heat storage capacity: 10^6 J) and continuous monitoring of the anode loading by the system software during operation limits anode roughening to such a minute level that changes in the beam quality due to increased inherent filtration by the anode cause no serious disturbance.

Furthermore, the probability that this effect will occur can be further reduced by the selection of a relatively large effective target angle. The X-ray tube employed in the SOMATOM offers the highest output reserve of all tube types yet introduced in computed tomography. The effective target angle has the unusually large value of 12°, determined by the scanner construction. For a constant beam quality and exposure time, the dose reproducibility and thus the contribution of quantum noise to the image noise level is determined only by the stability of the X-ray tube current. This is guaranteed for SOMATOM by means of a tube current regulator, which sets the heater current so that the X-ray tube current is maintained at the desired value. A positive side effect of this regulation is – along with the output reserve mentioned – a long X-ray tube life.

For CT scanners with a fan-shaped beam and detector systems which rotate along with the tube, such as SOMATOM, ring-shaped artifacts characteristic of the system unavoidably occur if the differences in sensitivities of the individual data acquisition channels are not compensated adequately. A measurement in air (without any object in the beam path) is therefore performed several times a day in order to determine the sensitivities of the individual data acquisition channels automatically. These measurements then yield the corresponding correction factors. For SOMATOM, this calibration procedure is initiated at the push of a button and is finished in such a short time, such as during changing patients, that there is no interruption of the normal sequence of examinations.

The accuracy required for the electronics of CT systems is very demanding. In order to prevent errors in measurement arising from drifting of the operating point originally set, the data processing system for SOMATOM automatically calculates an "offset adjustment", following each registration of data measured from the projection of an X-ray pulse. This maintains the operating points of the individual data acquisition channels, yielding a 0 V output when no X-ray signal is present at the input.

1.7 Temporal Resolution

The temporal resolution is a measure of image quality which cannot be obtained directly from a computed tomogram. Its effect is more indirect, since the scan time influences

▷ the occurrence of motion artifacts
▷ the number of data available for image reconstruction
▷ the applied patient dose

SOMATOM provides scan times from 1.4 to 14 s, permitting individual adaptation of the scanning times to the medical examination required and the ability of the patient to cooperate.

In carrying out a series of CT scans, the scanning time and the scanning frequency are particularly important. In this regard, SOMATOM permits a maximum scanning frequency of 12 scans per minute, assuming a scan of 3.2 seconds. Additional improvement in temporal resolution is also possible through segmental reconstruction, i.e. the reconstruction of an image from data acquired over a projection range of 240° (see 3.2.3).

Outlook for the Future

Modern CT scanners such as SOMATOM offer scanning times between one and two seconds. These scanning times are very short compared with the length of time over which a patient can hold his breath, so that this is seldom a problem with CT images. Blurring caused by the heart beat or pulsating blood vessels is, however, more difficult to suppress. This would require scanning times on the order of 10 milliseconds. The instrumental data acquisition would then be vastly more complicated and, presumably, it would not be possible to obtain a satisfactory image, in view of the dose which would then be available. Nevertheless, as

Boyd has shown [5], such extremely rapid CT scanning systems are already technically feasible.

However, the essential question is whether they are meaningful, i.e. whether there are enough fields of application and indications for introducing such a system. It is possible to obtain information about rapid processes from a series of relatively slow CT scans, as the example of Cardio CT (a CT serial technique using image reconstruction based on ECG) shows (see 3.2.3). Reducing the CT scan times from several minutes to about ten seconds and finally to about one second represents enormous progress. On the other hand, it is questionable that the technical effort necessary to reduce the scanning time by another one or two orders of magnitude can be justified.

Literature

[1] Performance evaluation SOMATOM DR. Erlangen: Siemens AG 1985
[2] Altar, W.: Westinghouse research memorandum 60–94410–14–19
[3] Cohen, G.; Di Bianca, F.A.: The Use of Contrast-Detail-Dose Evaluation of Image Quality in a Computed Tomographic Scanner. Journal of Computer Assisted Tomography 3 (1979) pp. 189-195
[4] Linke, G.; Geyer, H.; Brunner, J.: Objektives Verfahren zur Bestimmung des Kontrast-Detail-Diagramms. Deutscher Röntgenkongreß, Vortrag Nr. 160, 1983
[5] Boyd, D.P.: Transmission computed tomography, in T.H. Newton, D.G. Potts, Ed., Radiology of the Skull and Brain, Vol. 5, pp. 4357-4371. St. Louis, Mosby Co. 1981

2 Technology of Computed Tomography

2.1 System Concept

Computed tomography has developed from a special neuroradiological procedure to a widely applied X-ray examination technique. A modern CT system must therefore be able to scan all body cross sections and offer a range of operating parameters suitable for widely different diagnostic procedures.

As already mentioned, CT scanners are found today in medium-sized and small hospitals, as well as in large clinics and private practices. These installation sites vary greatly in terms of organizational structure and types of patient.

Consequently, a system concept is required which offers the greatest flexibility in the configuration of the system – particulary in regard to data processing.

The operational characteristics of a CT system are determined principally by the:

▷ type of scanning apparatus
▷ arrangement and material of the detector system
▷ beam generating system
▷ data processing system, including software

The following sections will illustrate the characteristics of scanner types and the different designs suggested for the individual system components. It will then become clear that there are usually different alternatives possible and that the decision in favor of a particular alternative depends upon the relative importance of individual positive or negative aspects of the design. The concept of a CT system and its components cannot be based only on technical considerations; it must always strive to take into account the needs which its practical application dictates.

2.2 Basic Types

The CT systems offered on today's market can be classified according to four basic types [1] (Fig. 2.1):

a) translation-rotation scanners with only a few detectors per slice
b) fan-beam scanners with rotational motion only and revolving detectors (referred to in the following material as fan-beam scanners)

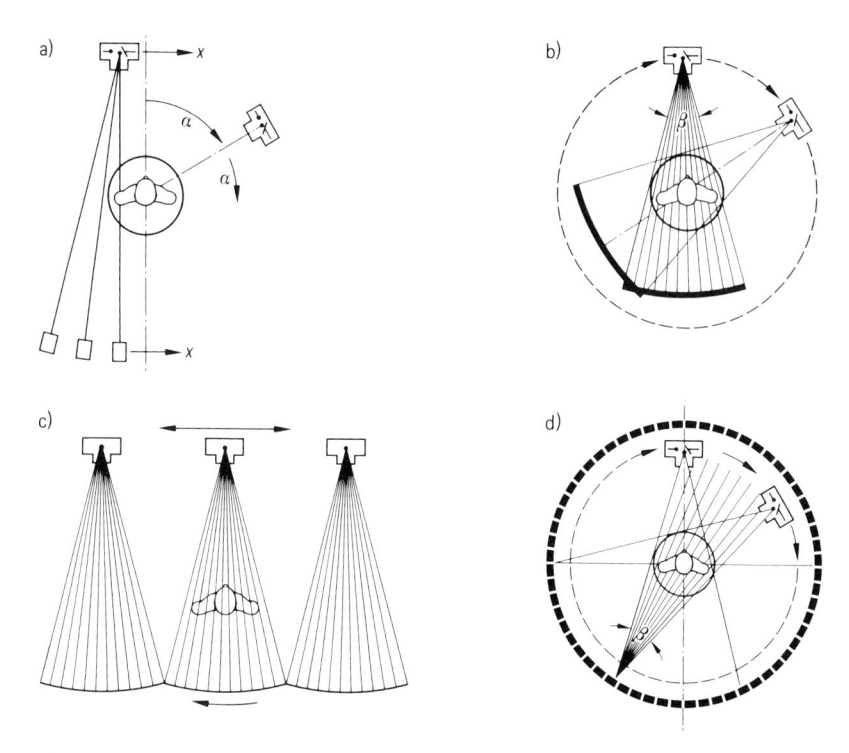

Fig. 2.1 Basic types of CT scanners

c) translation-rotation scanners with a large number of detectors, which therefore provide for the possibility of switching to rotation-only operation (referred to as hybrid systems)
d) fan-beam scanners with a stationary detector ring (referred to in the following as ring detector scanners)

2.2.1 Translation-rotation Systems

In terms of the motion which it describes, the translation-rotation scanner is the original CT scanner type [2]. However, in modern designs the main disadvantage of the original version has been largely avoided: the collimation of the X-rays to a single pencil-thin beam for each slice in the first CT scanners allowed the output of the X-ray tube to be utilized only over a tiny solid angle. As with the original CT scanners, a stationary anode X-ray tube serves as the beam source. Since it is cooled with water or oil, it has a relatively high long-term power rating of several kilowatts (long-term and peak power ratings being essentially identical). However, the complicated form of motion and the still relatively poor utilization of the beam output, in spite of the increase in the number of detectors, only permit scanning times in the range of a few minutes down to about ten seconds for translation-rotation scanners. This scanner type is therefore entirely suitable for standard head scans. For whole body scanning, however, where movement is to be expected, it is not altogether satisfactory.

2.2.2 Fan-beam Systems

Both types of fan-beam scanners function with a fan-beam which scans the entire object cross section. This design has the advantage of improved utilization of the radiation generated in the X-ray tube. Since the motion of the scanning system is uniform, rotating anode X-ray tubes with a substantially higher peak power rating of up to about 50 kW can be used in these scanners in place of stationary anode X-ray tubes. The higher short term power ratings of these tubes coupled with the uniform pattern of motion for these scanners permit scanning times of down to about one second.

2.2.3 Hybrid Systems

The hybrid scanner represents an attempt to consolidate the advantages of the translation-rotation scanner and the fan-beam scanner. On the one hand, the translation-rotation scanner offers good image quality along with inexpensive beam generation and inexpensive arrangement of detectors using relatively few elements. On the other hand, the rotating scanner offers very short scanning times, although this is at the expense of image quality (the available dose is low and the reduced number of detectors limits the spatial resolution) in the rotating mode of operation, if the system is to be kept simpler in design than a fan-beam scanner. A hybrid scanner can be described as a translation-rotation scanner with a somewhat extended range of application.

Summary

This brief discussion of scanner types serves to point out that, as a result of the shorter scanning times permitted, more efficient utilization of the X-ray tube output and the higher X-ray tube output available, fan-beam scanners are the more universally applicable systems and thus should be preferred over translation-roration systems.

2.3 Detector Arrangement

Deciding on the use of a fan-beam design is relatively easy. Deciding which of the two possible detector arrangements – stationary detector ring or rotating detector – both of which have been well developed for use in commercial scanners – is no longer so easy. Here the advantages and disadvantages of both systems, discussed below, must be carefully weighed in relation to each other.

2.3.1 Detector Geometry, Number of Detectors and Utilization of Dose

For the ring detector scanners, the number of detectors is determined primarily by the number of projections required to perform the image reconstruction (see 2.5). On the other hand, the number of scanning beams per projection can be selected by changing the ratio of sampling pulse frequency at the individual detectors and the angular velocity of the X-ray tube. For a fan-beam scanner (with rotating detector), the number of projections is independent of the number of detectors, which in fact corresponds to the number of scanning beams per projection. As a result of this difference, there are differences in resolution properties, in the number of detectors required and in the geometrical dose efficiency.

For the ring detector scanner, to attain the same geometrical resolution as with the fan-beam scanner generally requires more detector elements. The alternative would be to allow a considerable fraction of the radiation in the plane of the detector to go unused (Fig. 2.2).

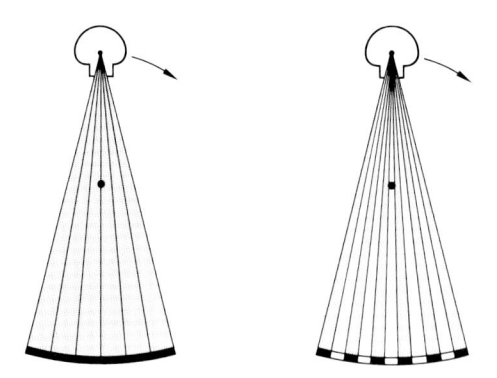

Fig. 2.2 Beam width and utilization of dose for a ring detector scanner

In order to achieve the beam width necessary for the desired level of resolution (see 1.2.2) the only recourse is to make the detectors narrower than the quotient of the detector ring circumference by the required number of projections. However, this would entail gaps between the individual elements, resulting in a loss of dose. With sufficient cost and effort, it is of course possible to eliminate these gaps through the use of additional detector elements and scanning more projections than are necessary. Another approach is to fill the detector ring with the desired number of wide detectors and provide the detectors with collimators which can be used to blacken out the elements in the azimuthal direction, thus reducing their effective widths in the interest of improving the resolution. This blackening out still does not fully utilize the beam which has passed through the patient. A third possibility to increase the resolution capability involves employing wide three-layer detector elements in the azimuthal direction, such that the two outer layers are chosen to be less sensitive than the middle layer. The beam is then utilized more efficiently, while an improved resolution capability also results. However, with such a configuration, the modulation transfer function characteristically falls off prematurely at mid-range frequencies in the diagnostically interesting region (Fig. 2.3) [3].

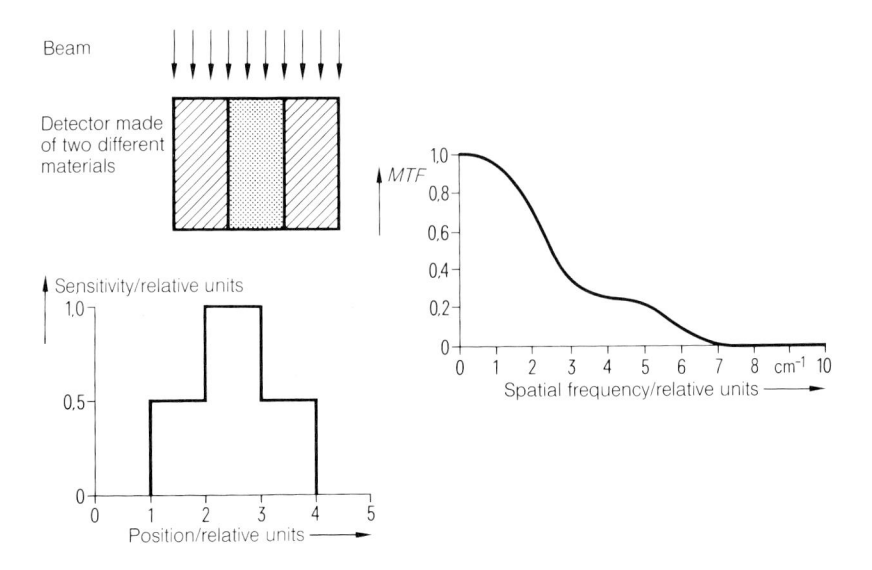

Fig. 2.3
Improving the resolution in a ring detector scanner through the use of detectors with non-uniform sensitivity in the azimuthal direction

2.3.2 Permissible Focal Spot Size

For classical ring detector systems, the X-ray tube rotates inside the detector ring. Consequently, for the same external scanner dimensions, the X-ray tube in the ring detector scanner is mounted closer to the axis of rotation than in the fan-beam scanner. The contribution of the focal spot dimensions to the beam width (see 1.2.2) is then greater for the ring detector scanner than for the fan-beam scanner. This implies in turn that, under otherwise identical conditions, a smaller focal spot with lower output must be used in the ring detector scanner.

One type of ring-detector scanner for which this limitation no longer applies employs a detector ring mounted inside the rotational path for the X-ray tube. It executes a nutation which is synchronized with the rotation of the X-ray tube (Fig. 2.4). This design has the disadvantage that, because of the nutation, the detector elements must be unusually long in the direction of the system axis and extremely homogeneous in their sensitivity over this entire length, a requirement which can be satisfied only with considerable difficulty. The detectors must also be arranged very close to the object scanned and therefore register a higher level of scattered radiation. This cannot be suppressed and is detrimental to the image quality.

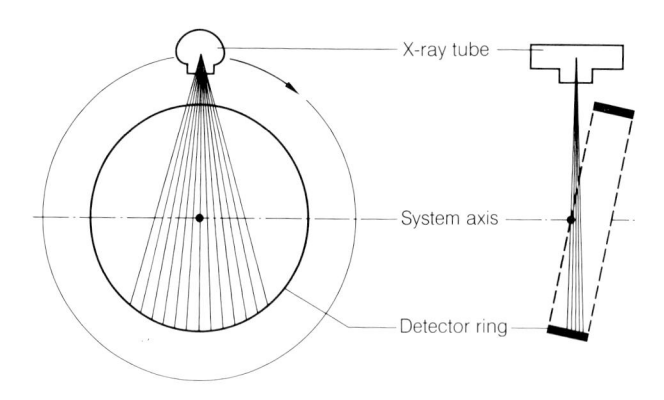

Fig. 2.4
Ring-detector scanner with nutational detector motion. This motion is synchronized with the rotation of the X-ray tube, enabling the tube to rotate outside of the detector array.

2.3.3 Collimation of Scattered Radiation

As in classical X-ray techniques, scattered radiation also worsens the quality of the CT image. If the detector system registers scattered radiation, this leads to the falsification of CT numbers during image reconstruction. These can only be corrected for very simple object forms, but not for the realistic case of a clinical examination. It is thus clear that any scattered radiation must be kept away from the detector system as well as possible (see 2.4.2).

In regard to the collimation of scattered radiation there are significant differences between the fan-beam scanner and the ring-detector scanner (Fig. 2.5). In the case of the fan-beam scanner, the useful part of the beam always impinges from the same direction on the individual detector elements. It is therefore possible to mount a very effective anti-scatter collimator, consisting of grids parallel to the axis and focussed on the focal spot, in front of the detector system. In the case of the ring-detector scanner, this is not possible. Due to the rotation of the X-ray tube, the useful part of the beam impinges on the individual detector elements from a constantly changing direction. The only possibility for attaining anti-scatter collimation comparable with that for the fan-beam scanner would be a collimator with moving grids aligning themselves automatically to the focal spot. The cost and effort required to develop such a device could not be justified. The only practicable way to reduce the scattered radiation signal for the ring detector scanner is to choose a large object to detector distance (Groedel technique) [4]. Under practical conditions, however, this method is far less effective than the collimator discussed above for the fan-beam scanner: in particular, it is totally inadequate for a ring-detector scanner with a nutation mechanism.

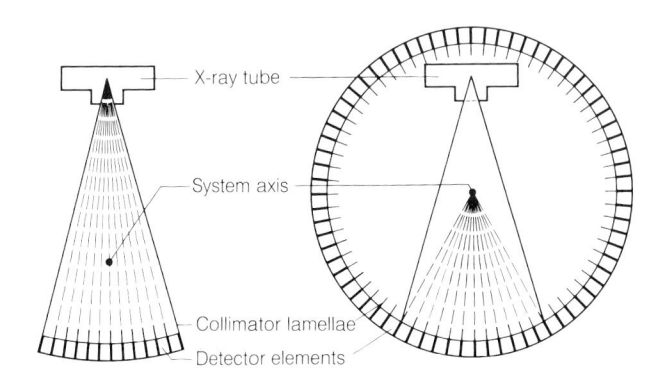

Fig. 2.5
Possible methods of collimating scattered radiation for the fan-beam scanner (left) and the ring-detector scanner (right)

2.3.4 Artifact Behavior

Another difference between the fan-beam scanner and the ring-detector scanner concerns the occurrence of artifacts caused by movements of the object during scanning. For the fan-beam scanner, the scanning time for one projection is between one and five milliseconds. For the ring detector scanner, the scanning time corresponds to the time required for the rotating anode X-ray tube to sweep over the fan angle; this is in the range of at least a tenth of a second. As a rule, then, the individual projections for the fan-beam scanner are not affected by object movements, and only object changes from projection to projection are registered. By contrast, for the ring detector scanner, there is a very high probability that disturbances caused by object motion occur even within the individual projections. This means that the same object motion gives rise to different artifacts for the fan-beam scanner and the ring-detector scanner.

2.3.5 Computed Radiography

For the localization of a slice as well as for many diagnostic procedures, a modern CT system must offer the possibility of computed radiography (CR) (see 3.1.1). More exactly, it must be possible to move the patient in the axial direction through the beam fan of the stationary CT scanning system registering projections at fixed distance intervals. These are then reproduced as for a conventional X-ray scan. This scanning technique is possible for both the fan-beam-scanner and the ring detector scanner. For geometric reasons, however, the ring-detector scanner generally employs less detectors in the CR fans than the fan-beam

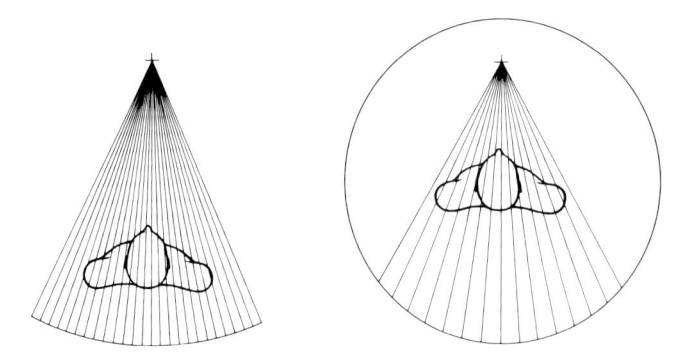

Fig. 2.6
Spatial resolution for computed radiography with a fan-beam scanner (left) and a ring-detector scanner (right) having a comparable number of detector elements

scanner. This means that the spatial resolution in the fan direction of the computed radiogram is lower for the ring-detector scanner than for the fan-beam scanner (Fig. 2.6).

2.3.6 Scanning Characteristics

In order to permit an image free of "aliasing" artifacts [5], the data acquisition must satisfy the Nyquist theorem: the distance between adjacent scanning beams must be no greater than half the beam width. The ring-detector scanner fulfils this condition easily, since the distance between the individual scanning strips can be easily adjusted by selection of the detector sampling time. By contrast, the fan-beam scanner has a fixed arrangement of beam widths and the scanning strips do not overlap, as the Nyquist theorem requires. A help here is the "quarter detector shift", i.e. installing the detector system so that the individual detector elements are displaced by one quarter of the detector element width and not situated symmetrically about the center line. Following a rotation of the scanning system through 180°, the rays from the shifted projections fall between the two adjacent rays from the opposite direction (Fig. 2.7).

For the same resolution capability, the fan-beam principle requires far less detector elements than the ring-detector principle. Without the quarter detector shift, it would even be possible to leave out one half of the detector arc (as long as the scanning system rotates through 360°, as in Fig. 2.8). This would permit a substantial reduction in costs.

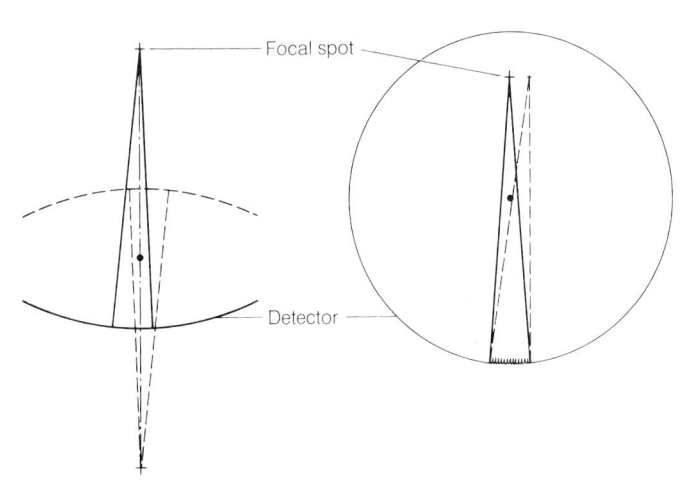

Fig. 2.7
Overlapping of scanning beams for the fan-beam scanner (left) and the ring-detector scanner (right)

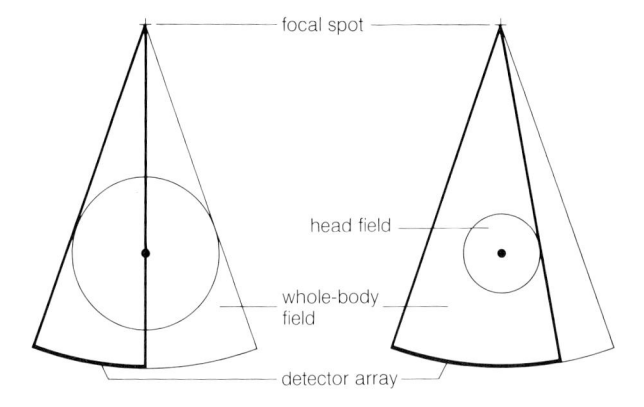

Fig. 2.8
Reduction in the number of detector channels for a fan-beam scanner. The example at the right shows the detector configuration for the SOMATOM DR 1.

On the other hand, for the same X-ray tube load, the effective image dose would be halved. However, ignoring the quarter detector shift would result in artifacts. Testing under practical conditions has shown that an altogether satisfactory compromise is possible (Fig. 2.8). This was implemented in the SOMATOM DR 1. The method utilizes the quarter detector shift and all the detector elements required for the (central) head scanning field. Only the detector elements outside of the head scanning field on one side of the detector arc are not used. Nevertheless, this means a saving of 25% of the detector elements and the associated electronics. For this, 25% of the total possible X-ray fan is lost by collimation, but a totally functional CT scanner remains: the absence of additional scanning beams does not produce artifacts in the whole body scanning field. Countless scans of the thorax and abdomen with SOMATOM DR 1 systems have confirmed this.

Summary

The relative importance accorded to individual characteristics determines whether the fan-beam scanner or the ring-detector scanner is to be preferred. It should however be pointed out that the fan-beam scanner is the system with the better dose utilization (for the same level of resolution and a comparable detector array), the better suppression of scattered radiation, the better resolution in a computed radiogram and the more flexible concept – particularly in regard to special applications, such as cardiac CT. For this reason, the two largest manufacturers of CT systems use the fan-beam priniciple.

2.4 Detector Types

2.4.1 Detector Construction

In fan-beam scanners, two different types of detectors are employed: high-pressure inert gas ionization chambers ("gas detectors") and scintillation crystals combined with light-sensitive semiconductors ("semiconductor detectors").

The *gas detector* (Fig. 2.9) consists of a pressure chamber in which the individual plate electrodes are mounted. The gas charge (usually xenon) is under a pressure of 10 to 20 bar. The length of the chamber is about 10 cm along the beam directions. The detector operates at a level between 500 and 1000 V.

The *semiconductor detector* (Fig. 2.10) is comprised of individual detector elements, each consisting of encapsuled scintillation crystals about 5 mm thick fixed

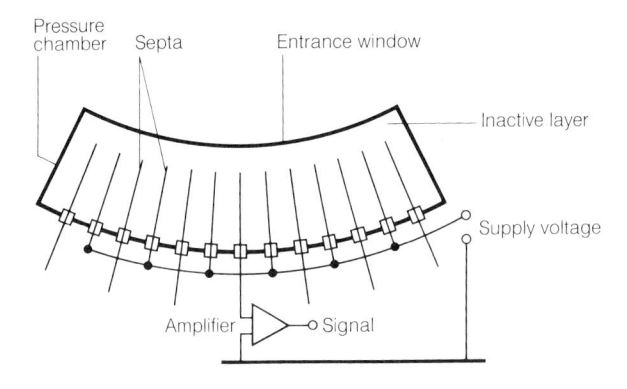

Fig. 2.9
Schematic of an inert gas detector. In a pressure chamber which is usually filled with xenon at 10 to 20 bar, the septa are insulated from each other.

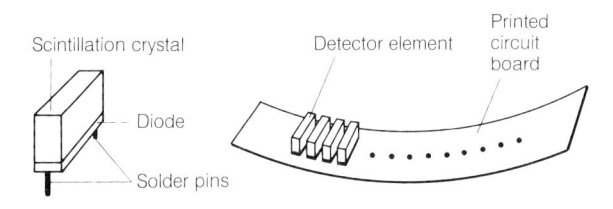

Fig. 2.10 Schematic of a solid state detector

to the surface of light-sensitive diodes. These individual elements are mounted on a printed circuit board. No special operating voltage is required.

Both detector types show characteristic behavior, which must be taken into account in operating a CT scanner.

2.4.2 Detector Characteristics

Signal decay

When scintillation crystals fluoresce as the result of impinging X-radiation, they continue to do so for a certain time following the incidence of the radiation. The physical constant describing this time is characteristic of the basic crystal material and its doping and can vary over several orders of magnitude [6]. For computed tomography, only materials having decay constants in the range of microseconds to milliseconds are of interest. Systems with a continuous X-ray beam (during rotation of the X-ray tube) require fluorescent material having a particularly short decay time. For an inert gas detector, by comparison, the decay constant is determined largely by the electrical circuitry.

Temperature dependence

The signal amplitude for some solid state detectors depends very strongly upon the operating temperature. Thus, for some detector systems, it is necessary to provide regulated heating or cooling in order to guarantee a stable detector output signal. On the other hand, for the inert gas detector there is no appreciable temperature dependence of the signal, because temperature changes give rise to a uniform change in pressure in all the chambers. Consequently, the surface density of the detector (gas mass per unit area) over the X-ray beam remains unaffected.

Noise and microphony

The inert gas detector has inherent sources of noise and disturbance not found with a solid state detector. Fluctuations in the voltage applied to the chamber can give rise to signal currents. The same is true for leakage currents in the insulating layer supporting the separating walls of the chamber. Due to its relatively large and thin plate electrodes, the inert gas detector tends toward microphony: the slightest shocks during operation can also generate a spurious signal.

The mechanical construction must therefore be carried out with great care.

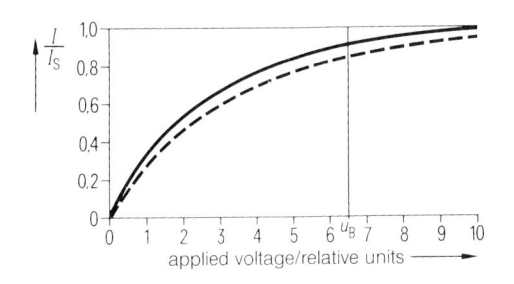

Fig. 2.11
Saturation effect in the inert gas detector

--- low dose rate
— high dose rate

Saturation effects

The range of linearity for a solid state detector, i.e. the region of characteristic operation in which the output signal amplitude is proportional to the X-ray amplitude at the input, extends well beyond the five orders of magnitude necessary for computed tomography. The inert gas detector, however, can show saturation effects over the same range of signal amplitude (Fig. 2.11). A well planned design (distance between separation walls, gas pressure and operating voltage) is required for the detector system in order to prevent such effects.

Anti-scatter collimation

There are no problems entailed in combining a scintillation detector with an anti-scatter collimator consisting of thin plates with a high attenuation coefficient, aligned toward the focal spot. This has been done with the SOMATOM detectors, for example. With most of the inert gas detectors for CT, special devices for scatter reduction are not used: the separating walls of the chamber serve simultaneously as anti-scatter collimators. Here, it should be pointed out that the effect of this arrangement is not as great as that of a separate collimator. Furthermore, somewhat more scattered radiation results from an inert gas detector than from a solid state detector. The principal causes of scattered radiation in an inert gas detector are the (due to the high gas pressure) thick entrance window (usually made of aluminum) and the layer of gas between this window and the upper edges of the plates.

Utilization of dose

For the usual crystal thicknesses of about five millimeters, the scintillation crystals used in computed tomography absorb practically 100% of the incident radiation and convert this into a light signal. For the solid state detector, no appreciable attenuating dead layers are required by the technology; for the inert gas detector, in which radiation leading to an output signal is absorbed both through the input window and in the layer of gas between the window and the upper edges of the plates, such layers are however altogether necessary.

Additional losses of radiation arise as a result of that part of the incident quanta (particularly with high energy) which pass through the detector without giving rise to an output signal. This effect can be limited to an acceptable level by the use of high gas pressures and chambers constructed as deeply as possible. From a mechanical standpoint, a carefully conceived manufacturing procedure is necessary in order to prevent the loss of gas, since even the smallest leaks will lead to a drop in pressure and therefore to an additional reduction in the absorption.

Summary

Just as for a consideration of the most suitable arrangement of the measuring components, the selection of detector type depends upon the importance accorded to the individual detector characteristics. Both types of detector discussed here are used in modern CT systems.

2.5 Generation of X-ray Beam

2.5.1 Beam Quality

In determining the scanning voltage for a CT system, it is always necessary to seek a compromise between the dose required for a CT image, the object contrast possible, the available X-ray tube output and the permissible patient dose. The voltage levels commonly used in computed tomography are generally between 90 and 140 kV. For small object diameters, the available dose permits working in the region of lower voltages and consequently in the region of slightly higher object contrast. This is at the cost of having to accept a higher patient dose for the same image dose than with higher voltages. Systems having low-output X-ray tubes demand the use of higher voltages at the cost of diminished object contrast.

Since SOMATOM is equipped with the CT X-ray tubes having the highest available output level, such compromises are entirely unnecessary. After careful consideration, the scanning voltage for normal operation was designed to be 125 kV. In addition to the inherent filtration resulting from 2.5 mm (aluminum equivalent), a 0.25 mm thick (or for the most recent model 0.4 mm) copper filter is also employed. This additional filter reduces the skin dose by more than 50% and at the same time reduces the detector signal amplitude only minimally. For certain special cases, SOMATOM provides the possibility of a lower voltage level, namely 96 kV, with identical filtration. Its use in clinical routine is rare, however.

2.5.2 Mode of X-ray Tube Operation

There are two possible modes of operating the X-ray tube for a fan-beam design: either the tube radiates continuously during its rotation and the measuring time for each projection is determined along with the number of projections by the sampling frequency from the individual detectors or the beam is pulsed, so that the pulse duration determines the time over which each projection is measured and the number of pulses per revolution determines the number of projections. For a given dose, the use of a continuous beam permits scanning at a lower peak load of the X-ray tube and the generator. The continuous beam method is thus of advantage if problems concerning the output and life of the tube would otherwise occur with the X-ray tube available. But this method also has disadvantages relative to a pulsed beam. As already mentioned in 1.2.2, during the scanning time the movement of the measuring apparatus contributes to the effective width of the strip measured and therefore to blurring also. In order to prevent unnecessary blurring due to movement of the measuring apparatus, it is thus necessary in continuous beam operation to select a large enough number of projections so that the distance which this apparatus travels between detector elements gives no perceptible contribution to blurring. For a given object diameter and limiting resolution – determined by the scanning geometry – only a limited number of projections is meaningful, however (Fig. 2.12). To reduce the contribution to blurring arising from movement of the measuring apparatus, the scanning of a larger number of projections may nonetheless be necessary.

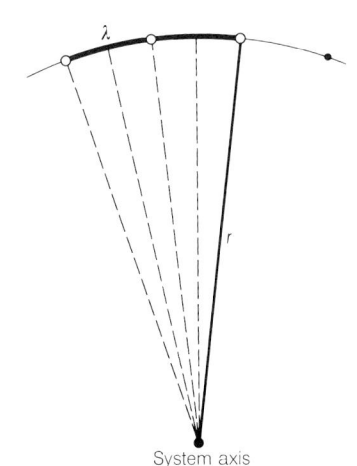

Distance between samples = ½ of periodic length

$$\frac{2\pi r}{N} = \frac{1}{2}\lambda$$

$$N = \frac{4\pi r}{\lambda}$$

Fig. 2.12
Required number of projections, N, for a fan-beam CT system

The Nyquist theorem requires that the azimuthal distance between scan beams is at most half as great as the periodic length of the smallest structure to be resolved

This also entails an unnecessarily high rate of data acquisition, a larger memory for these data and greater computational effort during image reconstruction.

SOMATOM uses a pulsed beam instead of a continuous beam for the following reasons:

▷ Pulsed operation allows defining a number of projections in agreement with the requirements determined by the object to be examined. In pulsed operation, the contribution to blurring arising from movement of the measuring apparatus can be controlled according to the pulse duration.

▷ As opposed to continuous beam operation, pulsed operation permits an automatic zeroing of the individual channels during the intervals between pulses. This precludes the falsification of signals due to drifting of the operating point in the electronics (owing to the necessary blackout, for continuous beam operation, such a zeroing would entail an unnecessary increase in the patient dose).

▷ For otherwise identical conditions the signal level in pulsed operation is higher, since the same dose is registered over a shorter time. This implies a more favorable signal-to-noise ratio in pulsed operation than in continuous operation, so that there is less noise in the images resulting, particularly for objects of large diameter.

▷ For pulsed operation (as opposed to continuous beam operation), it is possible with a suitable generator to switch between values of X-ray tube voltage between pulses, thus producing two scans at different beam energies during a single rotation of the measuring apparatus. This is an essential condition for effectively using the dual energy method, because this is the only possibility to guarantee the same geometry for both scans. If the two scans are run one after another, it is virtually impossible to avoid errors resulting from movement of the object under study (e.g., a different breathing position). With SOMATOM, the dual energy method switching is entirely possible by voltage levels between pulses (Fig. 2.13).

Pulsed operation with the high-output X-ray tube used in SOMATOM (OPTI 151 CT, heat storage capacity of the metal-graphite alloy anode 10^6 J) involves no compromises in regard to the life of the tube. The power rating of the rotating anode is so high that an anode rotational velocity of 50 or 60 Hz is sufficient for pulsed operation. This allows the use of high-tolerance bearings and guarantees a long life for the bearings in the rotating anode assembly. In the meantime, an X-ray tube with even better performance characteristics (OPTI 155 CT, heat storage capacity of the metal-graphite alloy anode 1.3×10^6 J) is now available for use in SOMATOM.

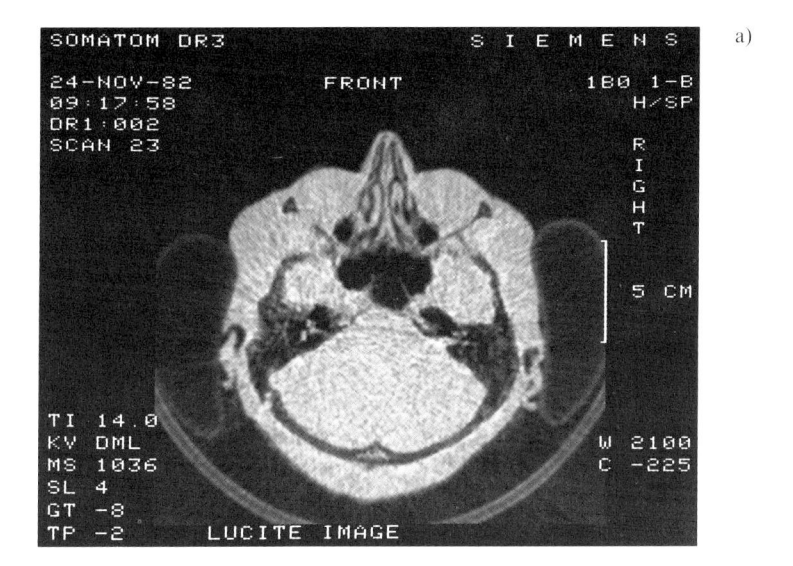

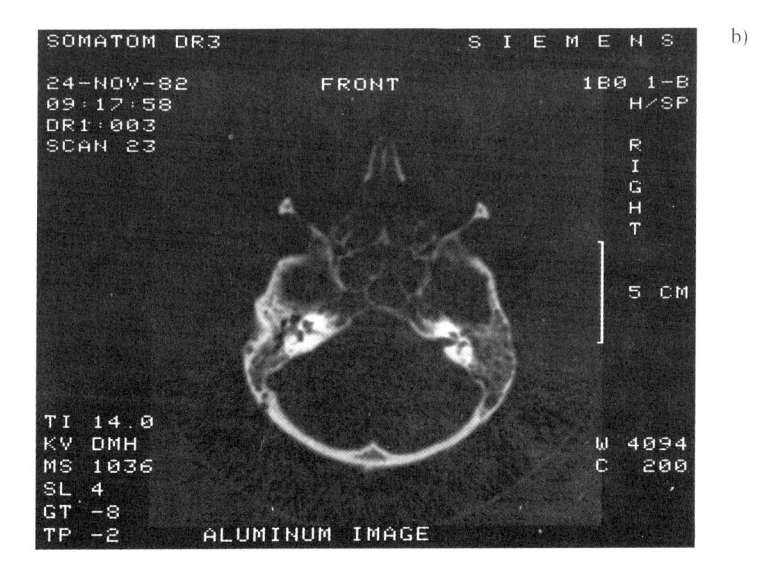

Fig. 2.13
Dual-energy method with switching of high voltage levels between pulses and computational analysis of object under study using two different basic materials: (a) plexiglas and (b) aluminum. The petrous bone artifact is much better defined in the standard scan (c) than in the dual-energy scan (d).

c)

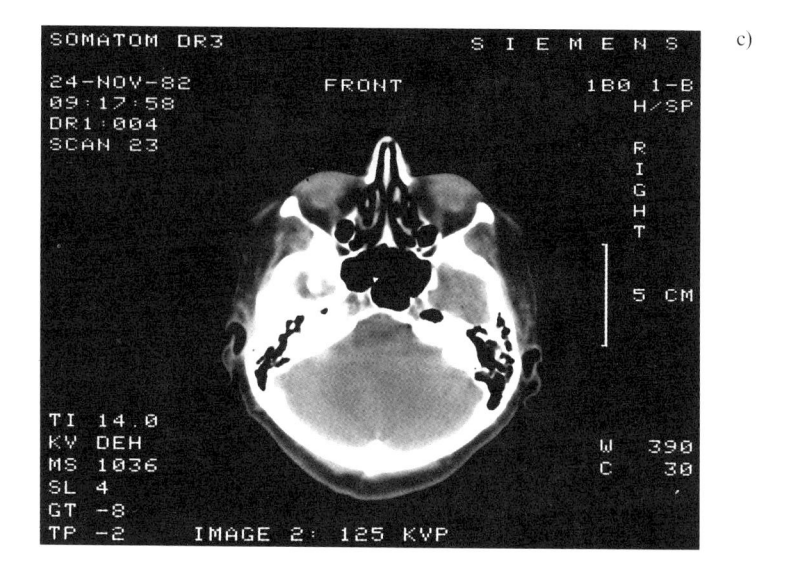

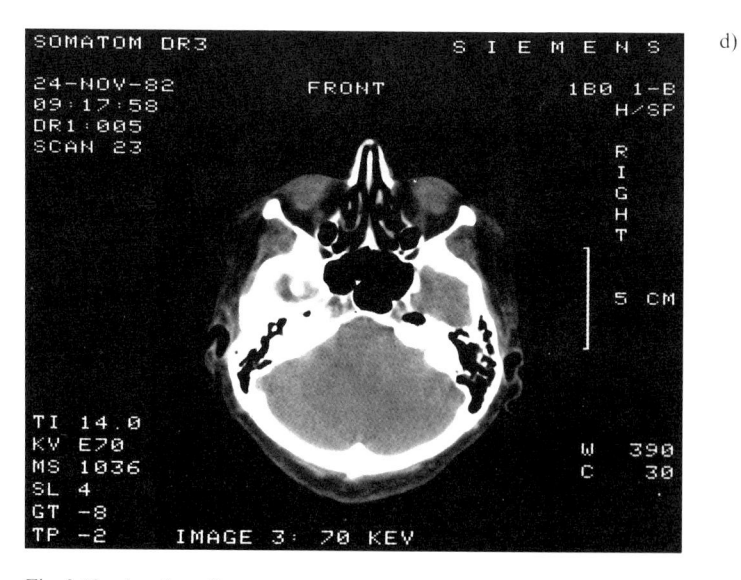

d)

Fig. 2.13 (continued)

2.6 Data Processing

2.6.1 Hardware

Electronics

The SOMATOM scanning electronics is designed especially for pulsed operation with solid state detectors (Fig. 2.14). A current-voltage converter, serving as input amplifier, and an integrator stage are connected to each detector element and perform the integration of the pre-amplified signal over each X-radiation pulse. In the intervals between radiation pulses, the signal at the output of the integrator is fed through multiplexing circuitry to an ADC and, following digitization, transmitted to the computer. Following each readout process the integrator is zeroed, so that the channel is ready to accept the next radiation pulse.

Along with the linear region for the solid state detector, which extends over approximately six orders of magnitude, a dynamic range of $1:10^6$ can be processed by the scanning electronics. This combination of characteristics permits the problem-free CT scanning even of objects having a large diameter (up to the scan field diameter of over 50 cm). Due to the wide dynamic range of the scanning system it is no longer necessary to use shaping filters to correct for object thickness in the peripheral regions. Therefore, it is not necessary to perform an individual beam hardening correction (see 1.5.2) in each channel or to seek a less complicated computer algorithm as a compromise solution for the beam hardening correction. Since no thickness compensation filter is used in SOMATOM, the resulting computed tomograms are characterized by outstanding homogeneity. This means that an object consisting of a homogeneous material is reproduced with a constant average CT number value over its entirety, and it is immaterial whether the phantom has been carefully centered or aligned eccentrically in the scan field (Fig. 2.15).

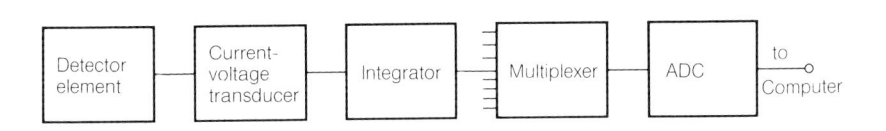

Fig. 2.14
SOMATOM scanning electronics (block circuit diagram)

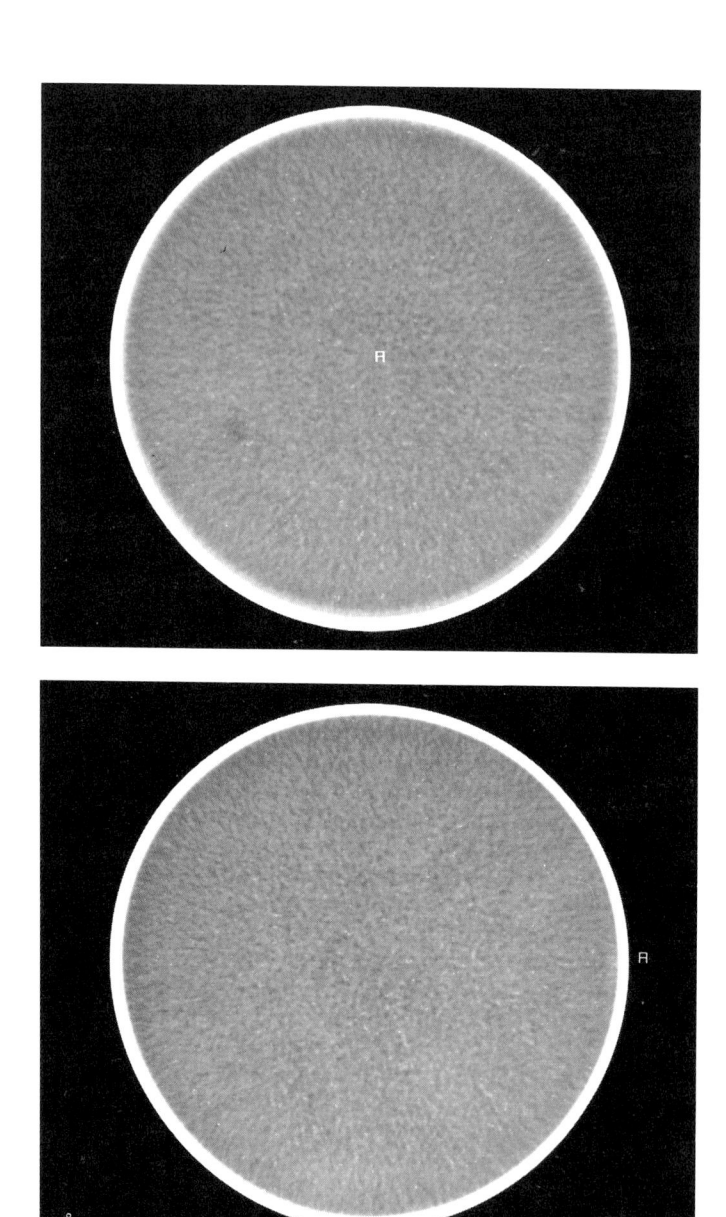

Fig. 2.15
Homogeneity of SOMATOM. A homogeneous object (water phantom) is reproduced with a constant average CT number value over its entirety, without regard to its location in the scanning field (above: centered, below: eccentric).

Computer

The computer in a modern CT system has a wide range of tasks to perform:

acquisition of scan data
image reconstruction
image display
image evaluation
image archiving

A computer capable of carrying out all of these tasks must offer both high-speed processing and flexibility, two characteristics difficult to reconcile with each other. For the SOMATOM computer system (Fig. 2.16), this is accomplished through the combination of a minicomputer known throughout the world (PDP 11/44 or PDP 11/24[1]) with our own BSP 11 fast programmable special computer.

The minicomputer is utilized as the host computer. It controls and monitors the system functions, coordinates the acquisition of data and the reconstruction of images and controls the peripheral data storage units (magnetic disc, diskette, magnetic tape).

The special computer reconstructs the image from the given scan data. The speed of computation is high enough so that the processing of the scan data keeps pace with the scan, yielding the finished image immediately following the scanning procedure.

Considering the large amount of data (up to 1,013,760 values for 704 scanning channels) and the high rate of data transfer (on the average about 1.5 Mbit/s), the demands made upon the minicomputer would greatly exceed its capabilities. Its bus, i.e. the signal transfer system connecting the central processing unit, memory and peripheral devices would not be able to provide data transfer in the short time required and its arithmetic unit would not be able to carry out the necessary operations over this time. For this purpose, a computer is required which is capable of operating on not only individual data, but entire fields of data (arrays), such as the entire scan data from a single projection, with a single command. The BSP 11 is such a special computer: it is an array processor tailored to the requirements imposed by image reconstruction from individual projections. It has its own bus system, connected through an interface with that of the host computer. This separate bus, to which the BSP 11 memory and arithmetic unit are connected, allows performing all necessary corrections on the scan data acquired by the computer, as well as convolution of the individual projections and finally back projection into the image reconstruction memory, without loading down the host computer bus.

---

[1]) Digital Equipment Corporation

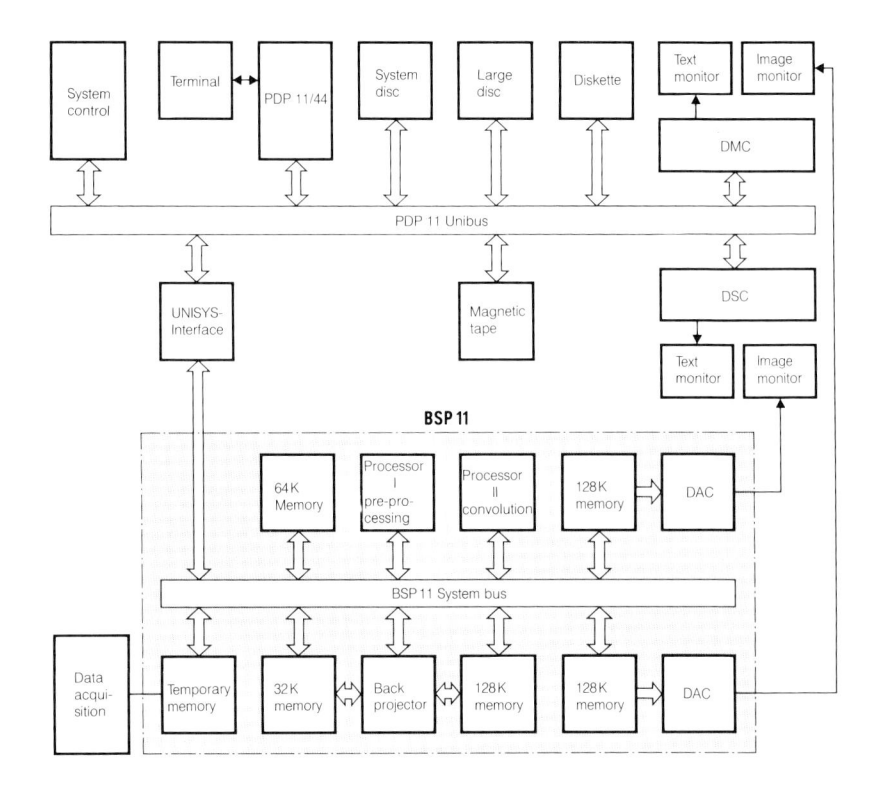

Fig. 2.16 SOMATOM data processing system (block diagram)

During the scanning procedure, only the pre-processed scan data are transmitted to the host computer bus for storage onto a magnetic disc. The performance characteristics of the arithmetic unit employed for pre-processing of scan data, convolution and back projection are chosen so that these three processing steps can be performed in accordance with the pipeline principle. In other words, while the data from one projection are being pre-processed, the previous projection undergoes convolution and the projection preceding this is back projected. This concept permits a rate of data processing which keeps pace with the scanning procedure.

Along with the arithmetic unit and memory capacity required for image reconstruction, the BSP 11 computer also includes the memory for outputting images as TV monitor displays, window settings for selecting the attenuation value regions of interest and digital to analog conversion.

The performance characteristics of the BSP 11 computer can be adapted easily to the task at hand through the use of another arithmetic unit and other memories. Thus, for the simpler versions of SOMATOM, only 256×256 and not 512×512 image matrices are provided for. Some users, however, find the image display from a 256 x 256 matrix too coarse. Consequently, it is possible by means of the appropriate hardware to interpolate this coarse matrix into a 512×512 matrix for display. This makes a better visual impression without having altered the information content in any way. Figure 2.17 demonstrates the display of the same object using three different matrices.

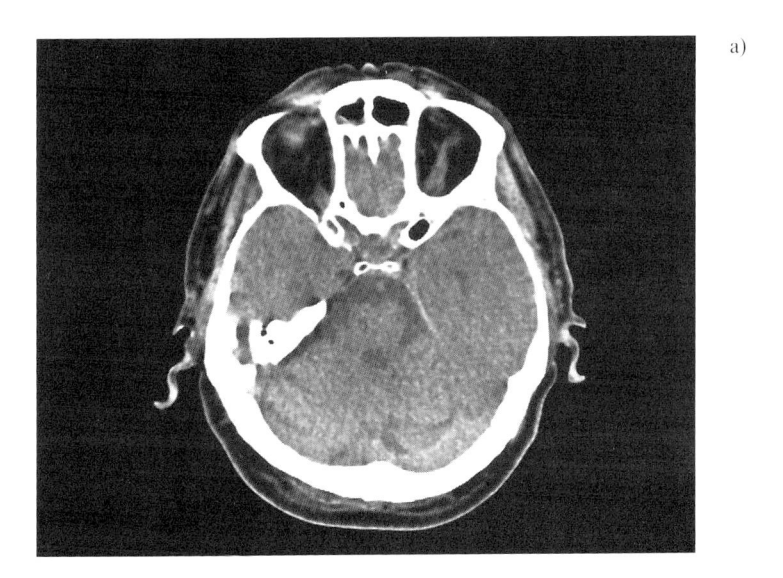

Fig. 2.17
Display of a single scan using three different matrices: (a) 512 × 512, (b) 256 × 256, (c) 512 × 512, interpolated from 256 × 256

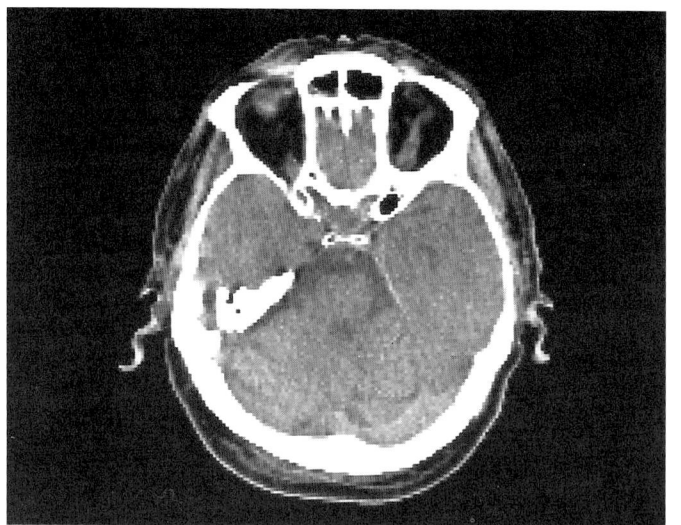

b)

c)

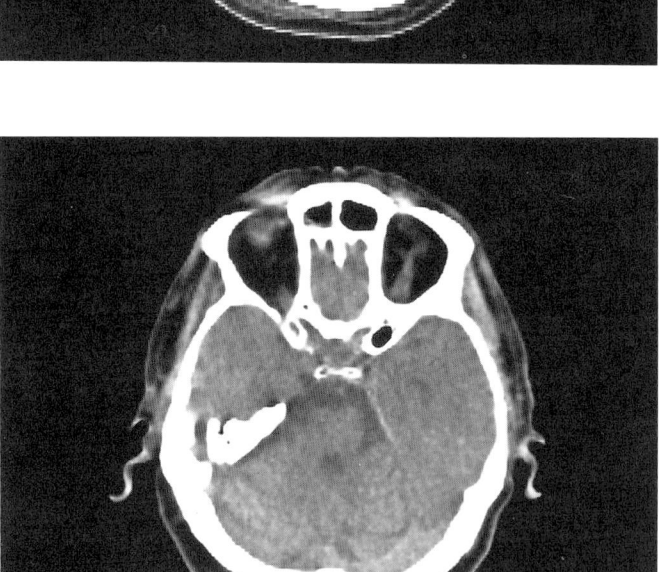

Fig. 2.17 (continued)

Control Console

The system is operated from the "diagnostic main console" (DMC, Fig. 2.18), which includes the dialog monitor and image monitor, as well as the input unit. Along with the usual typewriter keyboard, the input unit includes a large number of function keys and also a pen and resistor pad for inputting image positions. The main console is connected through an interface to the bus of the host computer. In addition to all necessary operating steps for scanning, it also performs all archiving functions – including photography – and calls up all image evaluation functions which SOMATOM offers.

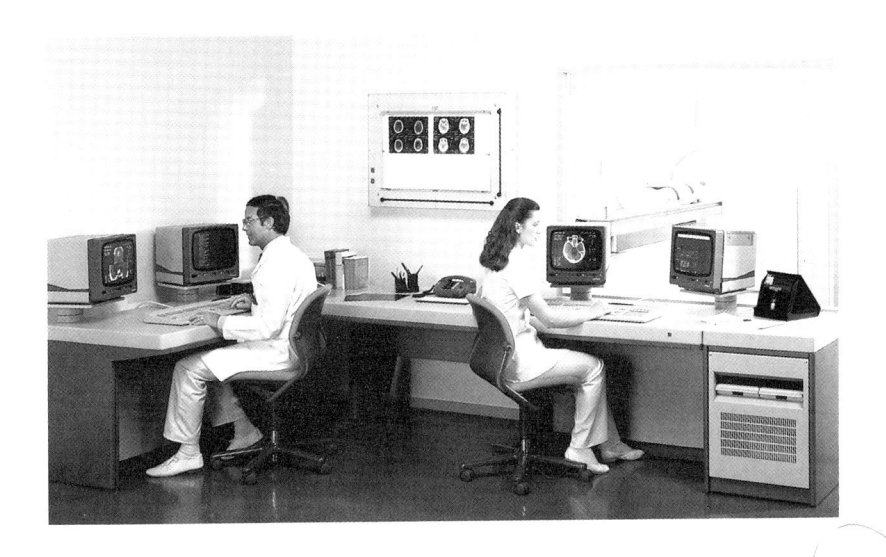

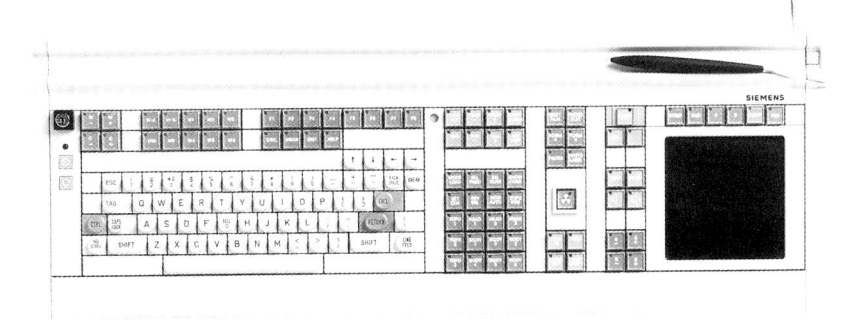

Fig. 2.18
SOMATOM main and diagnostic consoles (above) and their operating field (below)

Evaluation Console

Experience shows that image diagnosis tends to inhibit the rate of patient throughput, particularly when a large number of examinations must be performed. Therefore, the system can be equipped if necessary with an additional console, the diagnostic satellite console (DSC). In its appearance, it differs only slightly from the main console and is connected in the same way to the computer system. This type of diagnostic console offers the advantage, not possible with a workstation separated from the CT system computer, of being able to easily access all peripheral memory devices. It is also possible with the aid of the fast image reconstruction computer to reconstruct images in modified form from the diagnostic console, beginning with stored raw data. It is entirely possible to construct a completely independent workstation as desired from the appropriate system components.

Another possibility is to couple different systems together through a data network (e.g. ETHERNET or DECNET) in such a way that not only CT systems but also CT and MR units can be linked to each other. However, it is necessary to point out that this limits the rate of data transfer, so that it is only meaningful to transfer images between different devices.

Mass Storage Devices

The inclusion of a widely used standard computer as host computer permits using all mass storage devices available for this system (Fig. 2.19) with a minimum of effort to store images or raw data. Along with the dual diskette drive included in the basic SOMATOM configuration and a magnetic disc drive – for the newer systems, using Winchester technology with 2 x 25 Mbytes – it is also possible to connect magnetic disks having, at present, a capacity of up to 456 Mbytes. Such a disc suffices for 3300 scans with a 256 x 256 matrix, the number expected to accumulate over about one week. As soon as the new optical storage discs become available for the host computer system, they will be installed in SOMATOM. This will increase the memory capacity by at least a factor of two. Storage media having this capacity offer the advantage of being able to work very comfortably, but there is also the danger of losing a very large number of scans in the event of destruction or unintentional erasing of the memory.

Another inexpensive long-term archiving system offering an alternative to diskettes is a magnetic tape unit, which is available for SOMATOM. A tape having a length of 800 m can store 195 images, using a 256 x 256 matrix.

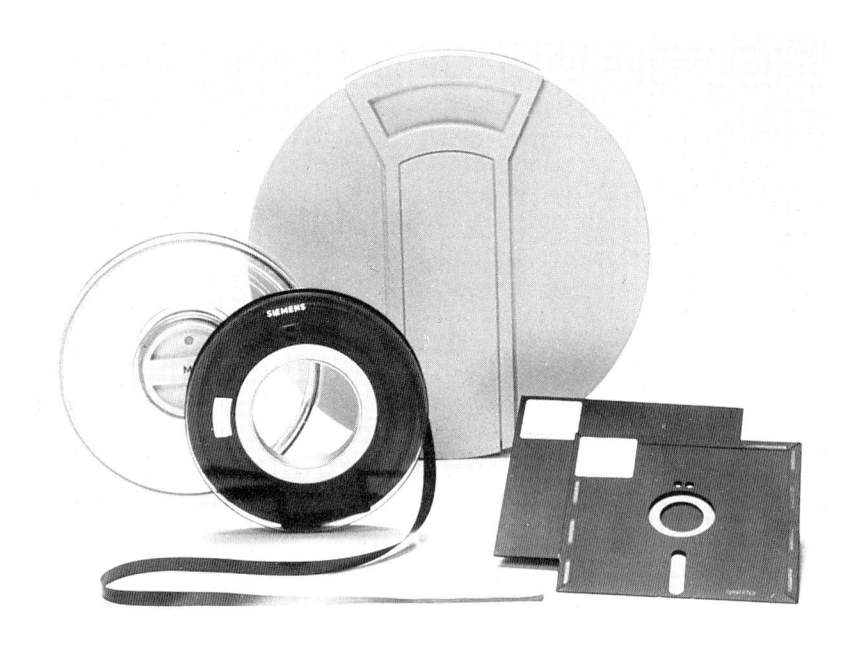

Fig. 2.19 Mass storage media for SOMATOM

2.6.2 Software

Operating System and Programming Language

The host computer is driven by the RT 11 x XM[1]) operating system. This operating system offers the possibility of expanding the memory beyond the 32 K words which can be directly addressed by the 16 bit machine as well as the possibility of foreground-background operation. This feature is used for the simultaneous connection of the DMC and the DSC: the operator's console runs in the foreground and the evaluation console in the background. The two consoles therefore make use of the available computing capacity by time sharing, the DMC having priority in order to guarantee that a scan can always be carried out to its conclusion without being delayed by commands initiated from the DSC. The software required for scanning, image evaluation, testing and adjusting the system is written in PDP 11 assembler, BSP 11 assembler or FORTRAN IV, according to the function performed.

---

[1]) Digital Equipment Corporation

The structure of the system operating commands is very similar to the commands for the operating system of the host computer: each command consists of three – in a few cases four – significant letters and can in general be supplemented by options also consisting of three letters, which are separated from the main command and from each other by slashes. In some cases, it is also necessary to provide information about the source and destination of information, as well as numbers identifying image or raw data sets. As an example, the command

COP/DAT DU 0:1 MS 0:

causes raw data set No. 1 from disc DU 0 to be copied onto magnetic tape MS 0. The number of the data set on the tape is not given, because the program automatically assigns these numbers in sequence.

Concept of operation

SOMATOM offers a wide range of scanning parameter combinations, for example two values for the X–ray tube voltage, seven different scan times including up to three mAs values and three or four different slice thicknesses. There are also many possibilities for image reconstruction parameters, for example eight convolution kernels, three high-resolution modes, various corrections for artifacts, zoom factors between 1 and 10 and an almost unlimited choice of reconstruction center. The possibilities for image evaluation functions cover a correspondingly wide range. Such a variety of possibilities could lead to problematical operation if no additional aids were present to simplify and abbreviate the dialog necessary for the selection of parameter combinations or evaluation functions:

▷ Function keys are provided for the permanent simplification of frequently required commands. Examples of these are
Scan start
Patient table advance
Standard archiving
Camera triggering
Image callup from temporary image storage
Setting windows
Determination of CT values
Selection of a circular scan area (ROI)
Measurement of distances and angles
Listing of the raw data and image data sets (directory) stored in a given memory
Callup of command list (help listing)

▷ The system user can define 16 scanning parameter sets of his own, which can then be called up as required by an abbreviated command without the need for further dialog. Some of these (three topogram parameter sentences and nine tomogram parameter sentences) can be called up by simply pressing a key

▷ Finally, both the DMC and the DSC are provided with eight function keys with which the user can program arbitrary command sequences. These can then be called up by activating the corresponding key. Each of these eight keys can be programmed up to four times, while the eight commands belonging to the group previously selected can be selected again by pressing a key and without having to enter any additional inputs. Thus, a total of 32 functions can be pre-programmed.

These provisions permit the nearly dialog-free operation of the system for standard examination procedures. As required, however, all possible combinations of parameters for scanning, image reconstruction and image evaluation which the system offers can be selected and utilized via dialog.

Scanning and image reconstruction

For every scan, the pre-processed raw data set is routinely stored onto the operating system disc, so that additional images – e.g. having a modified image character (convolution kernel, high resolution) or a different reconstruction center and imaging scale (zoom factor) – can be constructed as desired, until the data set is overwritten during the following scan. It is also possible, as required, to store all or certain selected raw data sets onto a magnetic disc assigned through the system, so that following an examination additional images can still be reconstructed. This can be initiated from the DSC without disturbing the scanning procedure.

Image evaluation

For the most important type of image evaluation, the selection of a limited region from the range of CT numbers in the image matrix for display on the monitor screen, eight function keys are provided in addition to the continuous window settings. Each of these keys can be programmed with two window settings, allowing the selecting of these windows by merely pressing the appropriate key. By combining one window setting from each of these two groups, it is very simple to arrive at a double window. Each window – including those selected by pressing a key – can be altered at will. A particular simplification for the operator is the possibility for automatically setting the center of one of the programmable windows to the average CT number at any location in the display by means of the pen and resistor pad.

The characteristic curve according to which the CT numbers are converted into brightness values can be varied at will and can therefore be adapted to the characteristic curve of the film material used, for example.

Apart from programmable window settings, SOMATOM offers numerous other functions for the evaluation and manipulation of images, among them:

> Measurement of CT numbers at any location in the image
> Printout of CT numbers from the selected image region
> CT number profiles along any direction in the image
> Measurement of distances and angles
> Computation of areas and volumes
> Statistical analysis of CT numbers within regions of interest (ROIs), for which rectangular, circular and elliptical ROIs are available along with the possibility to draw an ROI of any arbitrary form – up to three ROIs can be stored simultaneously
> Frequency distributions of CT numbers within the ROIs
> Mirroring of an ROI about any line in the image
> Mirror image of original image
> Image rotation
> Image enlargement
> Multiple image display
> Addition of images
> Subtraction of images
> Image filtering (with ten different filtering functions – see Fig. 2.20)
> Computation of secondary slices from scan sequences, for which any flat and even curvilinear cuts are possible.

Display of a scan series in such a rapid sequence as to give the impression of a film.

The possibilities which the SOMATOM software offers for evaluation satisfy practically every need. In the event that the user still finds it necessary to write additional diagnostic programs of his own, he can then fall back upon the USRLIB software option. This subroutine library permits addressing the image display memory, the function keys on the consoles and the pen and resistor pad from programs written in FORTRAN IV. It also includes routines for the callup and storage of images and for graphing on the monitor screen.

All necessary functions for the evaluation of computed radiograms ("topograms") are also available. The topograms can be utilized to interactively depict up to three body sections to be examined, for the automatic positioning of the patient table and for the determination of the angle of inclination required for the scanning unit (e.g. for spinal tomograms). Following CT scanning, it is possible to mark the slices scanned, including the applicable sequential number in the topogram (Fig. 2.21).

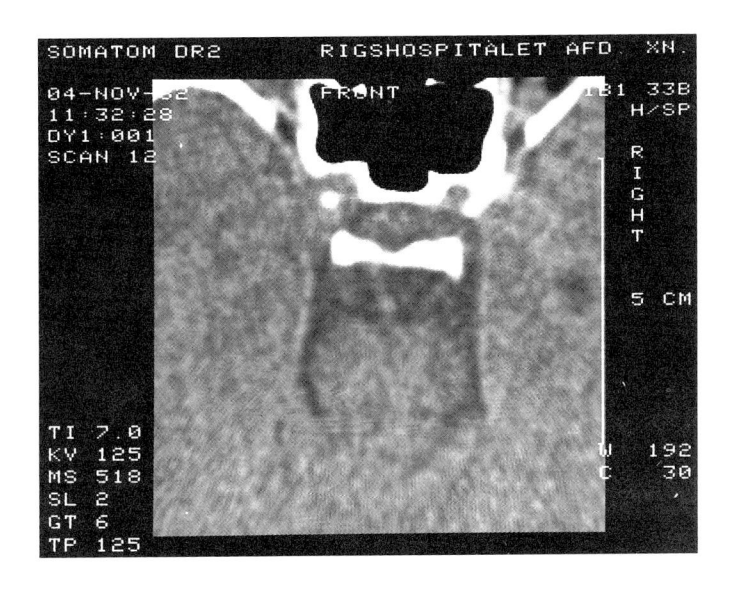

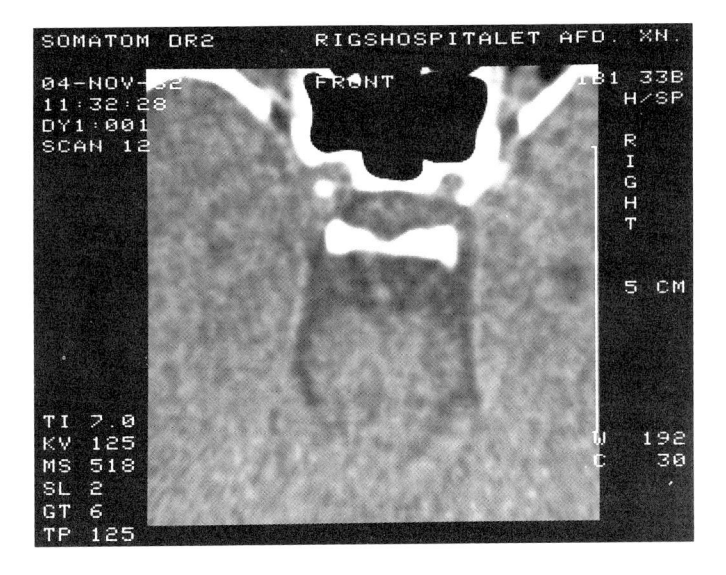

Fig. 2.20
Image filtering as an example of a SOMATOM image processing function

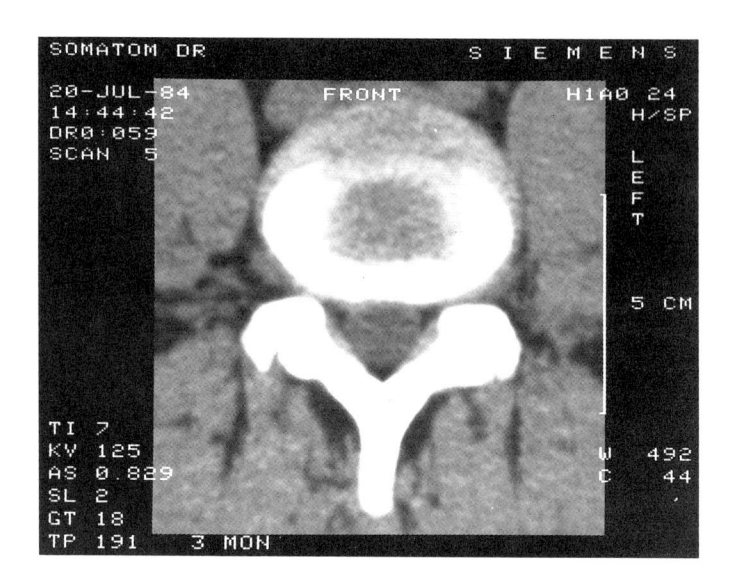

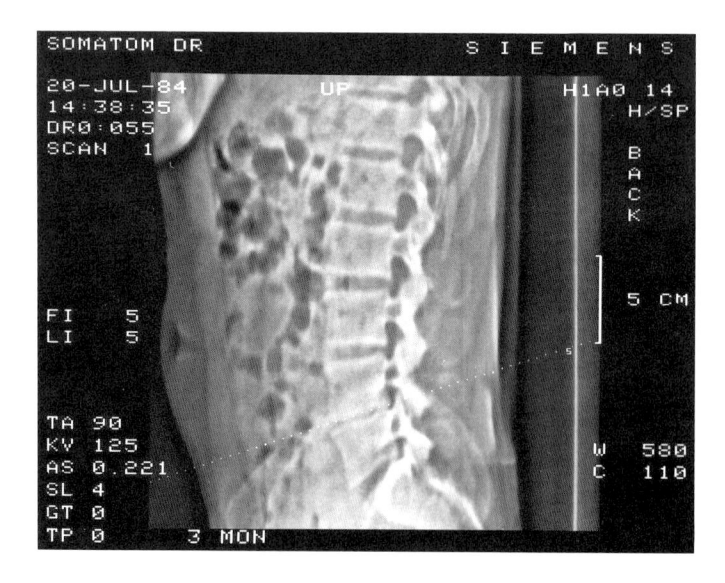

Fig. 2.21
Orientation of a tomogram (above) demonstrated with the aid of a topogram (below)

Archiving

For recording images on film SOMATOM offers the MULTISPOT M multiformat magazine camera, which is fully integrated into the CT data processing system. It can be controlled through the system software and can therefore be employed for fully automated documentation (after inputting the necessary command sequence). The 24 cm x 30 cm film format used can produce a large-format image or be divided into either four or nine images in smaller format.

For archiving onto magnetic storage media, SOMATOM offers diskettes or magnetic tapes. For reasons of cost, magnetic discs generally serve only for the temporary storage of images and CT data. For the archiving of image data, there are four modes of operation for SOMATOM: storage is in the form of either a 512 x 512 matrix or a 256 x 256 matrix and may be compressed or uncompressed. For uncompressed data, each image point is stored as an entire word, just as for the image reconstruction. Including the four header blocks, the data sets are then either 1028 or 260 blocks (each 256 words) long. For compressed data, this representation no longer applies and every odd-numbered CT value is stored as an even number (i.e. one bit information depth is discarded). This is still possible without a perceptible loss of image quality. Data compression reduces the length of the image data sets drastically, to about one third of their uncompressed length. The actual length of a compressed data set depends upon the content of the image, so that only approximate or average values are possible here.

Usually it is sufficient to archive images in the form of compressed 256 x 256 matrices. One side of an 8½" diskette (double density) is then able to store about ten images. A 10½" magnetic tape having a length of 800 m can store up to 600 scans under the same conditions.

Which of these two media is the more suitable for a particular user depends first on questions of cost and second on the frequency for accessing images previously archived. Diskettes are without doubt the more expensive of the two. However, search times on diskettes are only a small fraction of those on magnetic tapes. Consequently, the magnetic tape should only be used as an archiving medium when it is not necessary to access archived images very often.

Raw data sets can also be archived, but only in uncompressed form. Owing to the length of data sets (up to 4323 blocks), only a magnetic tape can be used here as the archiving medium. Since as a rule raw data sets are archived only very seldomly, the search and readout times on the magnetic tape do not present a serious limitation.

The archiving procedure requires only minimal effort on the part of the operator. After requesting archiving for a given sequence of images with a single command, it is only necessary to turn over the diskette or change the tape when called for by the program, in case no further data sets can be transferred to that diskette side or tape.

Literature

[1] Linke, G.: Technische Grundlagen der Computertomographie. Röntgenpraxis 30 (1977), pp. 159–180
[2] Hounsfield, G. N.; Ambrose, J.; Perry, J. et al.: Computerized transverse axial scanning (tomography). British Journal of Radiology 46 (1973), pp. 1016–1051
[3] Joseph, P. M.; Stockham, C. D.: The Influence of Modulation Transfer Function Shape on Computed Tomographic Image Quality. Radiology 145 (1982), pp. 179–185
[4] Groedel, F. M.; Wachter, R.: Unter welchen Voraussetzungen ist die röntgenologische Qualitätsdiagnose der Lungentuberkulose praktisch möglich? Beiträge zur Klinik der Tuberkulose und spezifischen Tuberkulose-Forschung 69 (1928), pp. 192–208
[5] Brooks, R. A.; Glover, G. H.; Talbert, A. J.; Eisner, R. L.; Di Bianca, F. A.: Aliasing: A Source of Streaks in Computed Tomograms. Journal of Computer Assisted Tomography 3 (1979), pp. 511–518
[6] Birks, J. B.: The Theory and Practice of Scintillation Counting. London: Pergamon Press 1967

3 Clinical Applications of CT Systems

The introductory chapters dealt first with criteria for the evaluation of CT scanning systems and their performance according to physical considerations and then at length with the possibilities for realization of the above requirements with present-day technology. The present chapter is concerned with the question of what additional physical and technical demands clinical practice imposes on a CT system. The relative importance of physical evaluation criteria should also be seen in this light.

The demands made upon the system and the relative importance of individual performance characteristics depend upon the user's requirements. The separate consideration in this chapter of routine applications, special applications and medical research takes this range of needs into account. Since routine application determines the overall concept, it is discussed first. This discussion is patterned after a routine scanning sequence. The really essential considerations will of course affect several areas of application to the same extent.

3.1 Aspects of Routine Applications

3.1.1 General Requirements for Operation of a CT System

The requirements imposed on the operation of a CT system stem from clinical routine and are well known. Operation should be simple and straightforward, requiring as few actions and as few dialog-oriented inputs as possible of the operating personnel and at the same time simplifying the necessary training. Since the scanner must be available at any time for emergencies, this is particularly important. In addition, operation of the system must be reliable. Since the CT scanner workstation is usually very much in demand, it is also desirable to have an ergonomically designed operating system.

It is of course difficult to respond to all of these requirements for each individual user. Consequently, it is necessary to offer a sufficiently flexible range of hardware and software to enable the user to help determine the operating concept. That there is a wide range of possibilities here will be seen in the following sections.

In general, it is necessary to set the requirement of simple and straightforward operation against the need to have a large number of scanning parameters, reconstruction parameters and diagnostic functions, all necessary in order to take full advantage of a modern CT system.

However, this should not force us to choose between a program of minimal capability running automatically at the touch of a button and uncomfortably complicated dialog operation. In fact, any operational sequence can be easily preprogrammed, so that an entire program sequence can be initiated at the touch of a button (see 2.6.2). The operator is free to define and store his own functions, which can then be performed with little effort or by relatively untrained personnel. These possibilities apply to the entire range of scanning commands and can thus be used in the selection of scanning parameters, as well as for diagnostic and archiving functions.

One possible ergonomic design for a workstation was already shown in Figure 2.18. The operator's console and the diagnostic console can be set up separately, but are both similar in terms of their operational concept. All operator functions and inputs are concentrated in a movable operator field, which can be repositioned to suit each individual operation. The function keys and scanning program keys are preprogrammed by the manufacture, but can be reprogrammed at will by the operator.

3.1.2 Patient Positioning

The range of patients which must be examined in computed tomography varies from a small child to a corpulent adult and must also include disabled and traumatized patients. The construction of a CT scanner must aim to provide as simple and secure a positioning as possible for all of these patients. In order to be able to scan the slices of interest without problems, a suitable patient table, a large scanning field, a gantry which can be inclined and suitable guides for positioning are all necessary.

There are numerous positioning aids available. In many difficult cases, it is advantageous to position the patient carefully outside of the examination room, provided that a patient transfer system is available (Fig. 3.1 a). Positioning aids are necessary in order to comfortably place the patient onto the table in the position desired and at the same time limit his movements as well as possible.

The selection of CT slices to be examined is entirely at the discretion of the operator. Deviations from the transaxial slice, such as for spinal examinations or as often required for studies of the base of the skull, are only possible with certain limitations. The greatest degree of flexibility is achieved with a gantry which can be inclined in both directions, used along with such suitable positioning aids as movable holding devices for the head.

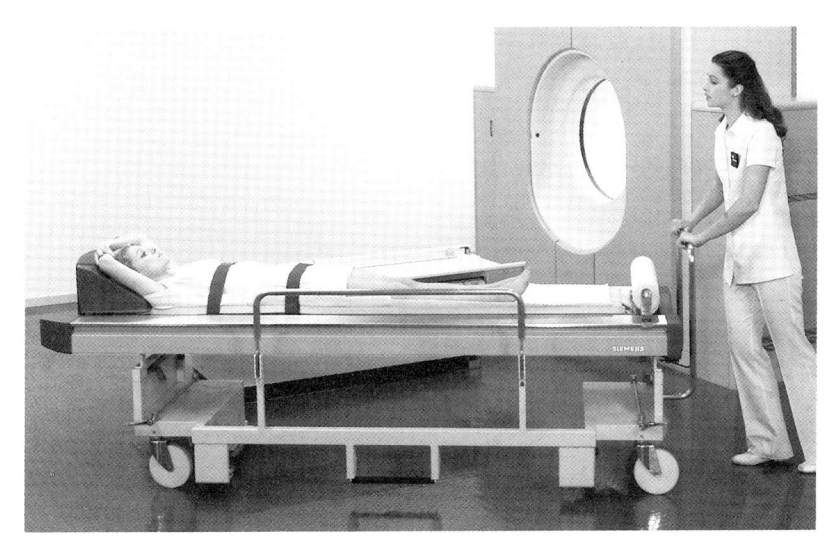

a) In difficult cases, the patient transfer system permits positioning the patient carefully onto the examination table outside of the examination room

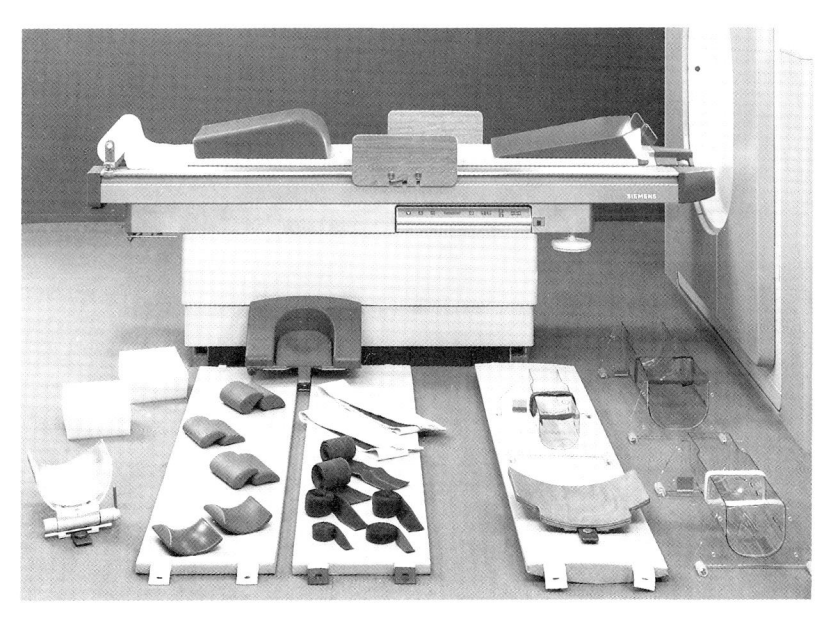

b) Numerous positioning aids are available for making the patient comfortable and limiting his movements. Baby cradles in various sizes serve to safely position infants.

Fig. 3.1   Patient positioning aids

Furthermore, the scanning field and the gantry aperture should have as large a radius as possible (Fig. 3.2). The larger the scanning field, the less is the danger that artifacts or CT value distortions will result from parts of the body outside the scanning field (see 1.5.5).

Patient positioning can be performed either by using the indicator lights or by means of a digital survey scan. The survey scan has proven to be a very useful means of positioning, particularly when high accuracy is required. It permits the exact selection of entire regions for examination and thus a fast-sequence automated examination (Fig. 3.3). Along with this, it offers additional advantages in terms of diagnosis and documentation (see below). Modern CT systems provide a positioning accuracy of a few tenths of a millimeter. Survey scans can be performed from various angular directions, with SOMATOM for any given tube position from 0 to 359°.

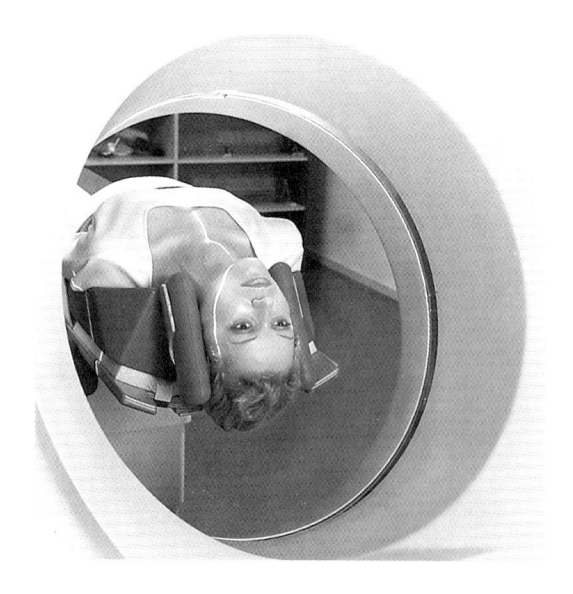

Fig. 3.2
Direct coronal slice orientation with a swiveling holding device for the head and a gantry inclination of 25 degrees

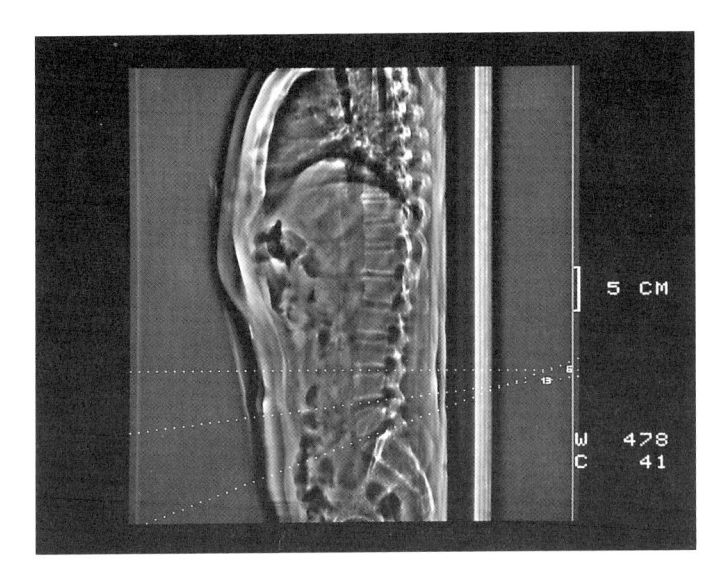

Fig. 3.3
Lateral topogram of the spine. The survey scan serves to determine the optimum gantry inclination and to position the patient exactly. Several regions of examination can be preselected.

3.1.3 Selection of Scanning Parameters and Flexibility of the Examination Procedure

For a given clinical procedure, the examination sequence is determined largely by the ease of operation of the CT system (see above) and the available scanning parameters. The most important scanning parameters are:
▷ the scanning time and scanning frequency
▷ the dose (mAs)
▷ the slice thickness

The selection of one parameter affects selection of the others.

With modern scanners, scanning times can be selected down to 1 second, while the range of standard scanning times is from 2 to 7 seconds. As a rule, when an extremely good image quality is required, particularly in regard to resolution, longer scanning times are necessary, since a higher dose is required. This is only possible over a longer time, because the output of every X-ray tube is limited.

The same consideration also applies to the scanning frequency. An arbitrarily rapid sequence of slices over a longer time is possible only with a low dose. Even then, the limit is determined by the loading capacity of the X-ray tube. The importance of the performance capabilities of these system components for the fastest possible routine operation cannot be emphasized enough.

The selection of the dose, which is directly proportional to the mAs value (the product of X-ray tube current in milliamperes and scanning time in seconds), must then be matched to the scanning times and scanning frequencies. The required settings for all of these parameters of course depend upon the degree of obesity and skeletal structure of the patient. Up to 500 mAs should be available for routine operation.

The selection of slice thickness depends upon the region examined and the nature of the examination. Thick slices permit a rapid examination procedure, while thin slices may be necessary when stringent requirements are imposed on the spatial resolution and the avoidance of partial volume artifacts.

The possible selection of different high-voltage values is also frequently offered, but in practice this is seldom used. Usually only one standard value is used, which is recommended by the manufacturer based on a consideration of the prepatient filtering and the detector. The optimum dose utilization and as low a patient dose as possible are the primary considerations (see 2.5.1). Using different kV values for different applications can however prove advantageous. In fact, it is absolutely essential for dual-energy CT methods.

3.1.4 Image Reconstruction and Diagnosis

The necessary computer time is the decisive parameter for image reconstruction. Without a doubt, it is desirable to be able to view the image by the time the scan is completed (instantaneous image). The importance of the instantaneous image or, equivalently, of very short computation times, can be understood from a number of points of view. From the standpoint of the operator, no one operating a CT scanner wishes to wait for the computer to reconstruct and display the image. Viewed from a cost-effectiveness standpoint, faster computation times generally imply a faster examination sequence and consequently a higher patient throughput. The decisive considerations are however to be found in the conduct of the examination and patient safety. The result of the examination in progress should be available at any time. The immediate control of the image following each scan is then optimal, in order to determine if the scanning parameters were correct and the image reconstruction was optimal (Fig. 3.4), as well as whether the region examined should be extended or the examination terminated.

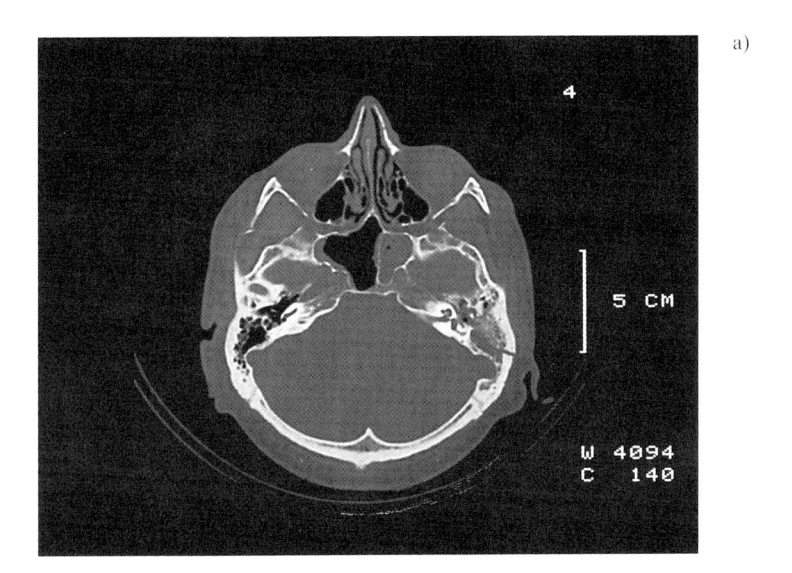

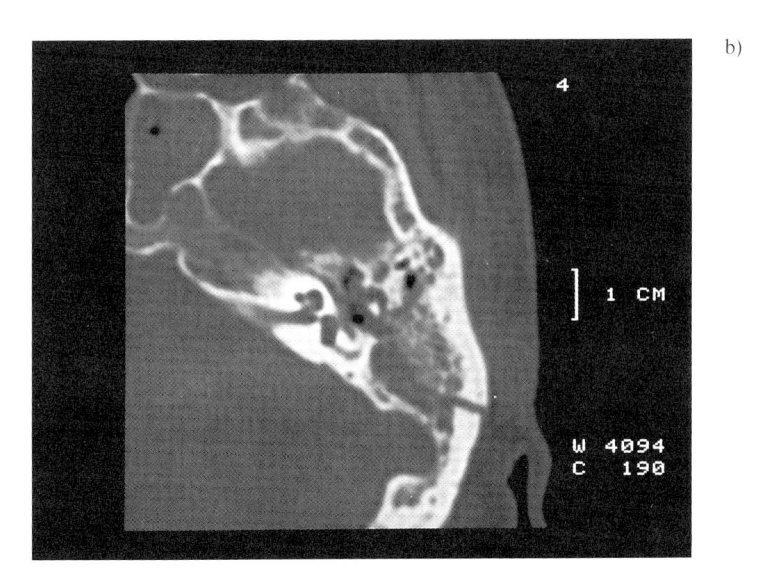

Fig. 3.4
Instantaneous images can be selected for any given reconstruction parameters: (a, c) normal reconstruction, (b) eccentric zoom in high-resolution mode, (d) eccentric zoom with normal reconstruction

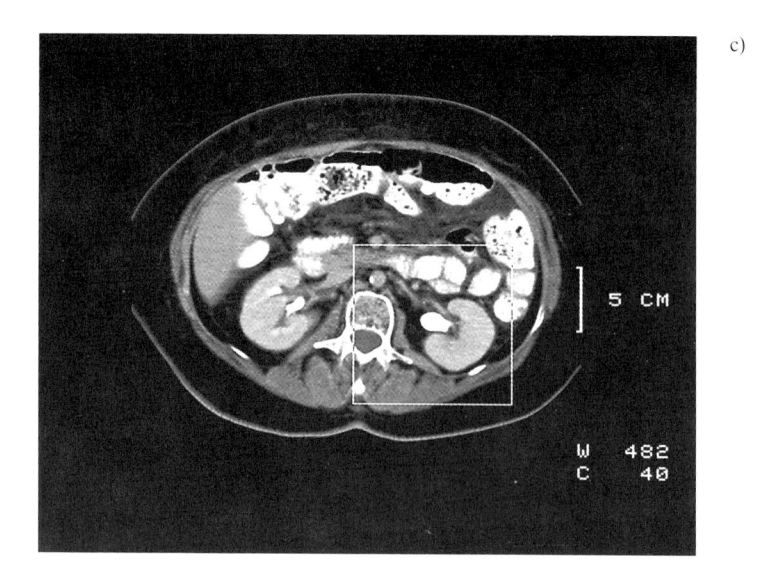

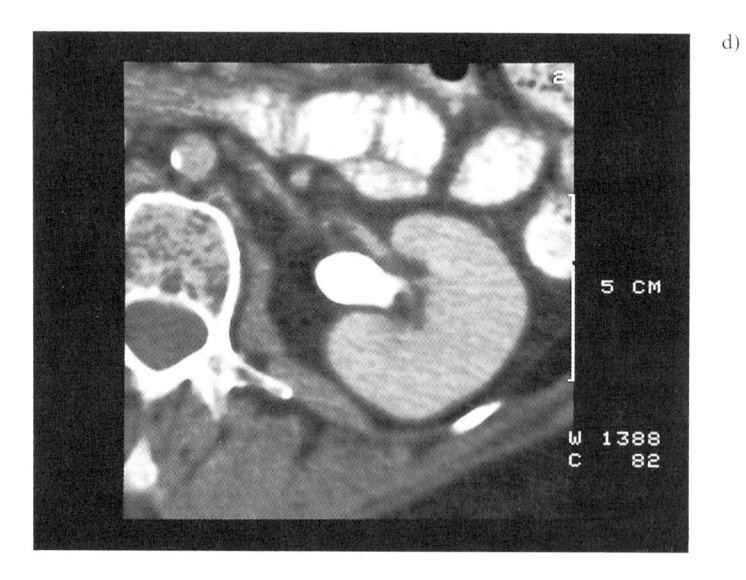

Fig. 3.4 (continued)

This is especially important for uncooperative or traumatized patients and when a contrast medium is used. Scanning without reference to the image can result in unnecessary strain on the patient from scanning irrelevant slices. Even worse, it can lead to having to scan additional slices after the patient has been moved from the examination room.

The diagnosis of CT images from the monitor screen is very often preferable to film diagnoses and is supported by numerous software functions (see 2.6.2). The diagnostic functions range from the acquisition of density values through simple geometric parameters, such as distance and angle, to statistical functions. All of these are gaining in importance, particularly for special applications (see below). There are also more extensive diagnostic functions, which permit synthesizing new images from stored image data. For routine applications, mainly the generation of reformatted images (Fig. 3.5) and the transfer of lesion contours into the

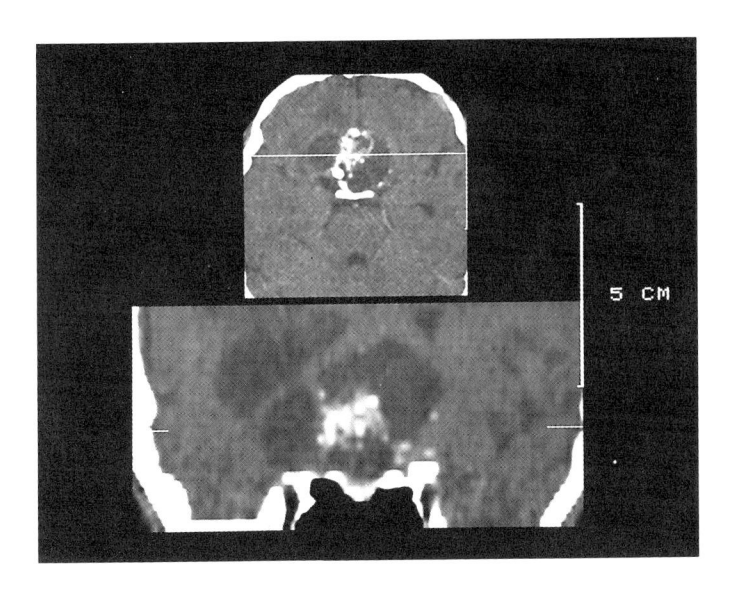

Fig. 3.5
Secondary image reconstructions. Any desired additional images can be calculated from the primary transaxial scan (upper half of figure). The example in the lower half of the figure shows a coronal slice through the pituitary region.

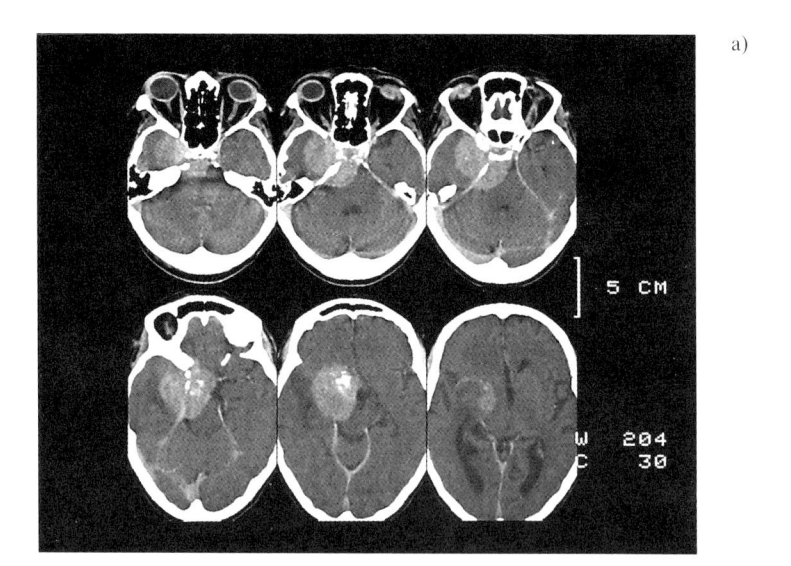

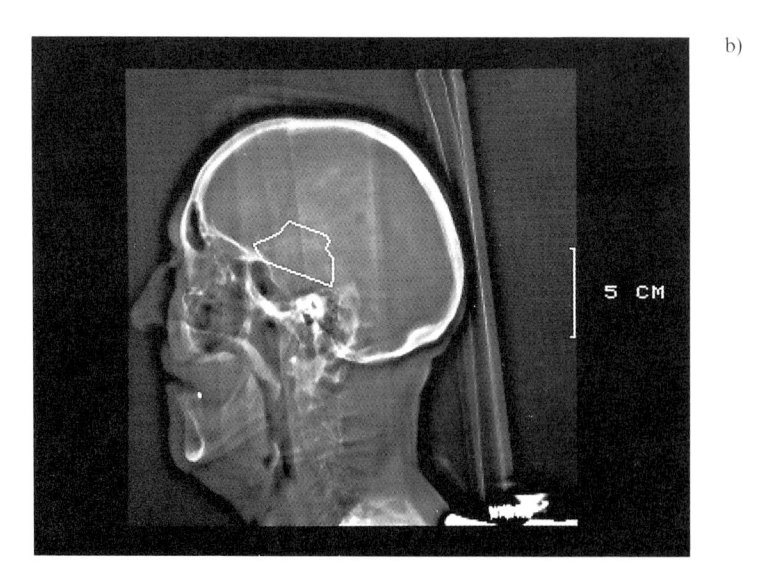

Fig. 3.6
Information from the CT image can be transferred to the survey scan image. The contours of a lesion made visible only through CT (a) are transferred for therapy planning to the lateral (b) and the AP topogram (c).

c)

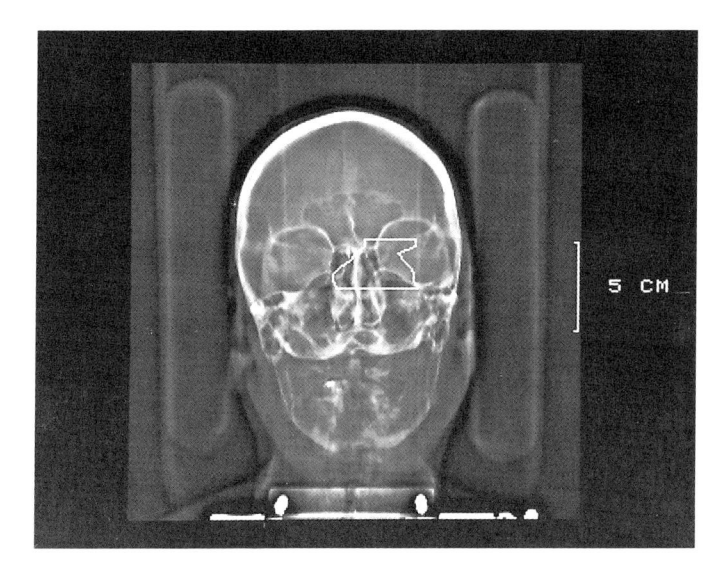

Fig. 3.6 (continued)

survey scan can be mentioned here (Fig. 3.6). Often, these supplementary images are of less value to the roentgenologist than they are to the surgeon or radiation therapist responsible for treating the patient.

Two main requirements emerge from the numerous and often-used possibilities for diagnosing images. In order not to limit or interfere with routine operation, diagnoses should be made at a separate console (Fig. 2.1.8). Often, this has the additional advantage that the roentgenologist can work undisturbed outside the control room. The other requirement is that the diagnostic functions must be performed with a minimum of computer time, if they are to be used routinely. It is then a great help if the required operational dialog sequences can be preprogrammed easily, so that they are initiated at the touch of a button. With SOMATOM, the operator has complete freedom to define and store his own functions.

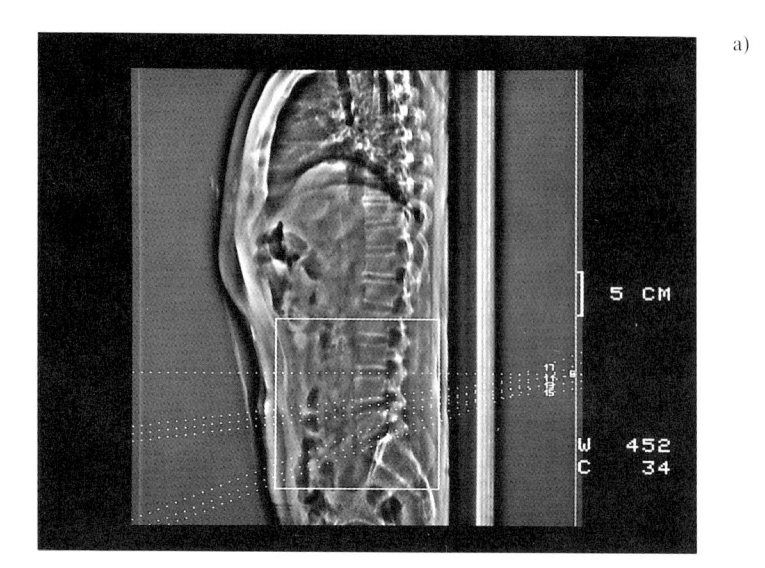

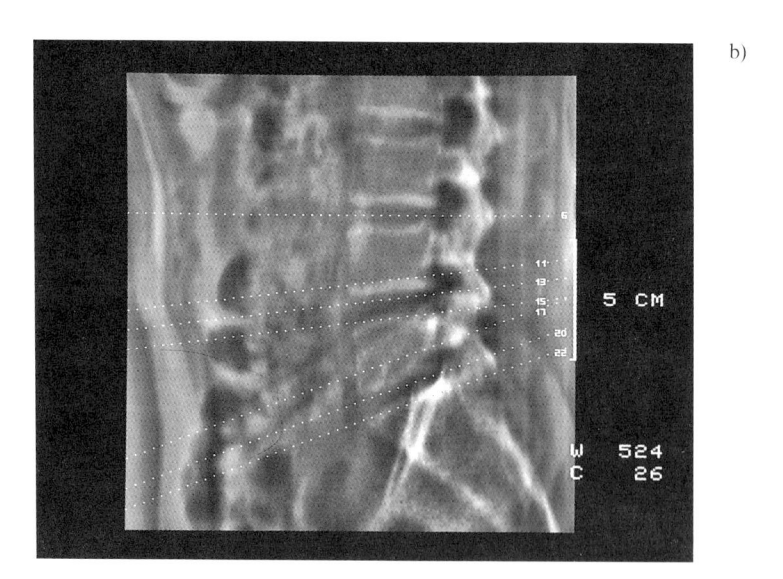

Fig. 3.7
The sequence of slices scanned is documented in the topogram in a clear and easy to follow form (a):
When a large number of slices is involved, a subsequent enlargement (b) permits greater ease in surveying the image

3.1.5 Image Documentation and Archiving

Documenting the findings from an examination and archiving the resulting images require a substantial part of the time for routine operation. Consequently, all measures which reduce the time needed for these tasks are worthy of particular consideration. In practice, the photographic documentation and the archiving of digital images onto magnetic tape comprise the greatest part of this time.

Optical memory and PACS (Picture Archiving and Communication Systems) are not yet ready for routine operation.

At present, photographic documentation is certainly the safest type of long-term archiving. Multiformat cameras are available for archiving, which allow the almost arbitrary subdivision of the transparent film from large format to diapositive format. The task is made easier by software-controlled magazine cameras, such as the MULTISPOT M, supported fully by the SOMATOM software. Even the use of a film magazine already represents a simplification, since the frequent changing of film cassettes is then no longer necessary. It is possible, though, to automate the entire photographic procedure, taking into account in advance the desired representation of the image in regard to the window setting and gradation curves. The camera should in any event be operated from a central console.

The software offers still other functions to support documentation. Scanning data and patient data, diagnostic results, marker arrows and commentary can be overlayed onto the topogram, as well as marking the slices examined as an aid for orientation (Fig. 3.7). Gradation curves can be freely selected for the monitor or the film camera, permitting optimization of the image result.

Archiving of digital images onto magnetic storage media saves the entire information content. Image diagnosis functions and processing functions can be used again at any time, for example. Typical times for accessing memory may lead to intolerably long storage times. A simple solution is then to transfer the archiving procedure to the diagnostic console or to carry this out after all scanning has been performed for the day. This was discussed in greater detail in section 2.6.

3.2 Special Applications

Specialized procedures in CT were developed very early. A few of these, such as dynamic computed tomography, are now established methods that should be available on all CT systems available today. A number of other procedures are still being developed or clinically tested.

This section discusses the system characteristics which are decisive for attaining optimum results from such special applications. The requirements imposed on the CT system which are dictated by research problems and go beyond the possibilities intended by the manufacturer will be dealt with in the following section.

3.2.1 Optimizing Image Quality

The simplest example of a special application for computed tomography is that of optimizing the image quality for particular clinical applications. Such measures are frequently ignored, ostensibly because they exert intolerable strain on "routine operation" or because the CT system is incapable of realizing them. Examples are:

▷ thin slice techniques
▷ high-resolution CT
▷ high dose level techniques

The most important technical and physical aspects of these methods were already explained in Chapters 1 and 2. Their advantages and disadvantages in relation to their use in the clinic will be discussed here. The conditions under which the necessary time and the demands made on the operating personnel can be held to a minimum while at the same time permitting the routine optimization of image quality will now be formulated more precisely.

The Thin Slice Technique

The imaging of thin slices is necessary for the optimal recognition of fine details and also often for the suppression of partial volume artifacts. The spatial resolution perpendicular to the scanning slice is improved, while the voxels imaged become smaller and are thus better approximations to an ideal cube (see 1.2.5).

A well known example is the examination of the inner ear. However, the need to image thin slices is just as great for all examinations of the base of the skull and the orbits. Even for spinal examinations or orthopaedic procedures, such as imaging a joint, the thin slice technique is of diagnostic interest. An additional advantage is clearly the possibility of improving the quality of secondary reconstructions, as Figure 3.8 illustrates for the example of temporomandibular joint scans.

It should be mentioned that, with the thin slice technique, it is unavoidable that a larger number of slices is necessary to image the same region of examination. An increased patient dose is also necessary in order to achieve the same signal level as for wider slices, if low-contrast resolution is required. This means that the thin slice technique is only possible in routine operation with a fast scanning sequence and a high X-ray tube output. In order to be able to speak of a true thin slice technique, slices having optimized sensitivity profiles (see 1.2.5) of 1 to 2 mm must be available.

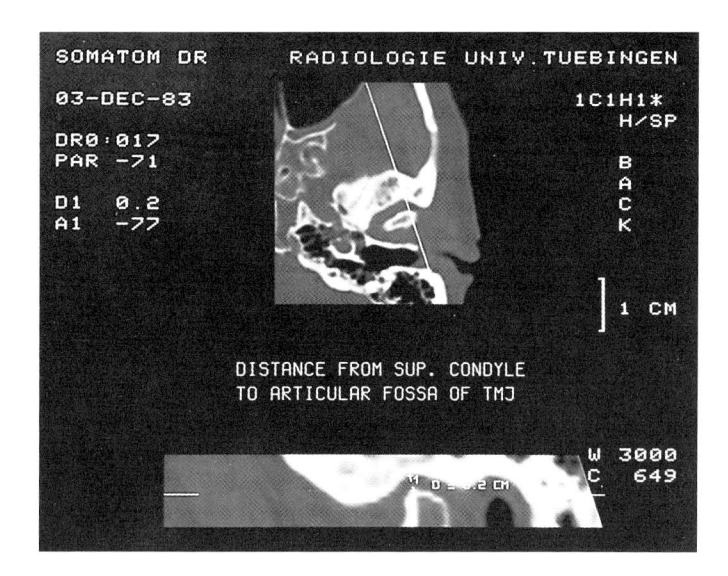

Fig. 3.8
High-resolution scans of the jaw using 1 mm slice thickness (above). This results in excellent secondary reconstructions (below). The distance between the upper functional surface of the condylus and the glenoid cavity can be determined exactly and is 0.2 cm.

High-resolution CT

High-resolution CT is understood to mean special methods of image reconstruction which take full advantage of the maximum spatial resolution possible with the given CT system. For a few types of scanners, the disadvantages for the operator are that intolerably long computation times are required or that the high-resolution CT images can only be reconstructed with special programs, after the examination is finished. High-resolution CT can only be employed routinely when the image reconstruction takes place during or immediately following the examination, i.e. when computation times are short. The SOMATOM offers this possibility: high-resolution CT images can even be selected and generated when scanning in the instantaneous image mode, with free selection of the zoom factor and the center of the region to be reconstructed (Fig. 3.9).

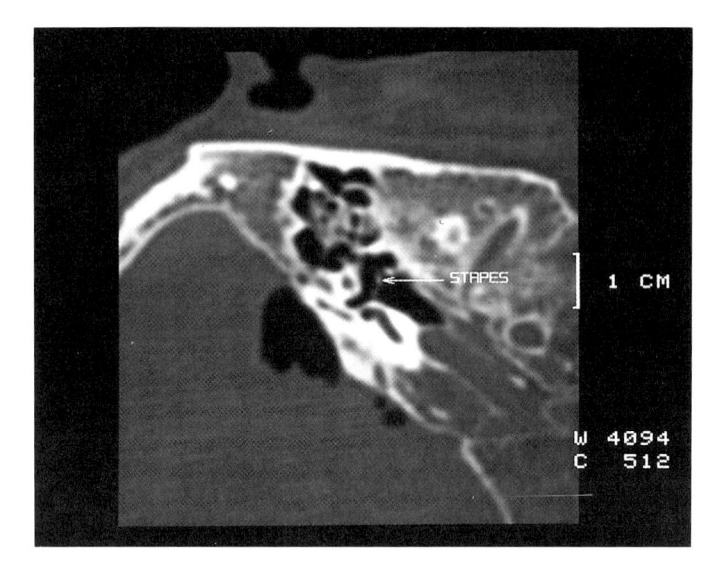

Fig. 3.9
High-resolution scan of the inner ear. The thin slice technique permits good images of even the stapes.

The High Dose Level Technique

The aim of the high dose level technique is the representation of very low contrast levels, such as in the central nervous system. Here, a high dose level is tantamount to a low noise level and a high level of contrast recognition. In order to take full advantage of the signal produced and to minimize the patient dose, a high-efficiency detector system is mandatory. For special applications, the CT scanner should offer values on the order of magnitude of 1000 mAs (Fig. 3.10). Relatively short examination times are possible only with high-performance X-ray tubes (SOMATOM, at 1036 mAs for example, permits 9 scans in 10 minutes with 0.1% (1 HU) contrast sensitivity, for 8 mm detail size, or 0.3% (3 HU) for 4 mm detail size).

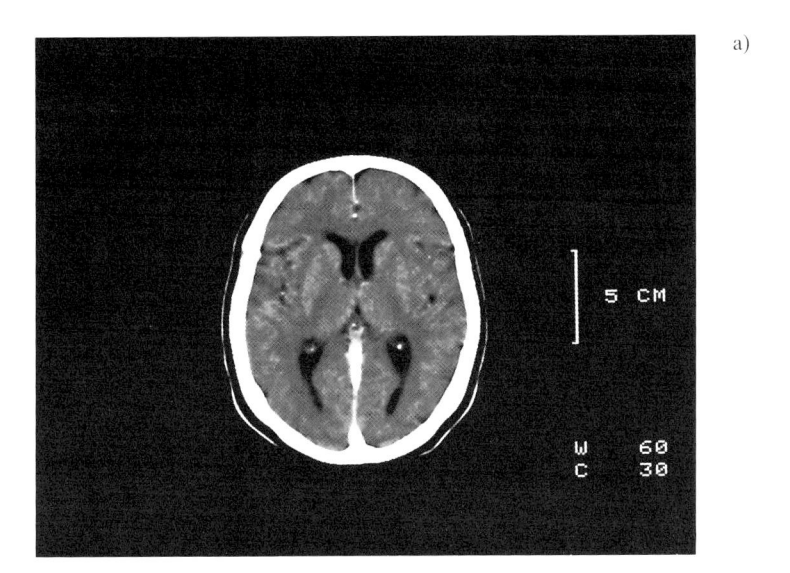

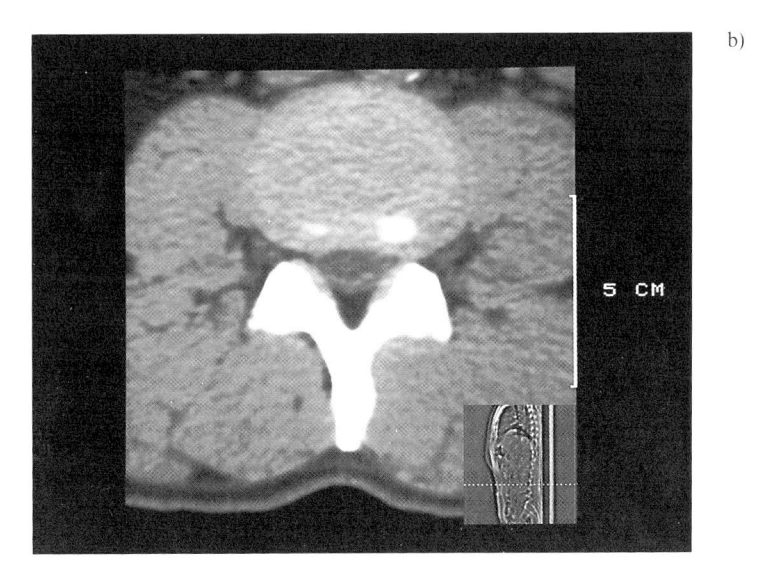

Fig. 3.10
High dose level CT scans (1036 mAs) permit the low-noise imaging of low contrast details in the brain (a) and the spinal canal (b)

3.2.2 Quantitative Computed Tomography

The CT image represents a remarkably good reproduction of an anatomical cross section. Along with this purely morphological information, in many cases sufficient for a diagnosis, the CT examination also yields quantitative information. The CT number values allow absolute and reproducible assessments of the density and, within limits, of the chemical composition for the body region examined. This quantitative information can be used, for example, to determine the mineral content of bones [1] or the fat content of the liver [2] (Fig. 3.11). In many cases, it permits assessments of the type or nature of a lesion [3]. A complete survey of the numerous applications and the extensive literature on this subject is beyond the scope of this book. In clinics where a suitably equipped CT system is available, CT number values are very often cited as additional information of relevance to the diagnosis. Quantitative computed tomography is however not yet established as a routine part of the examination.

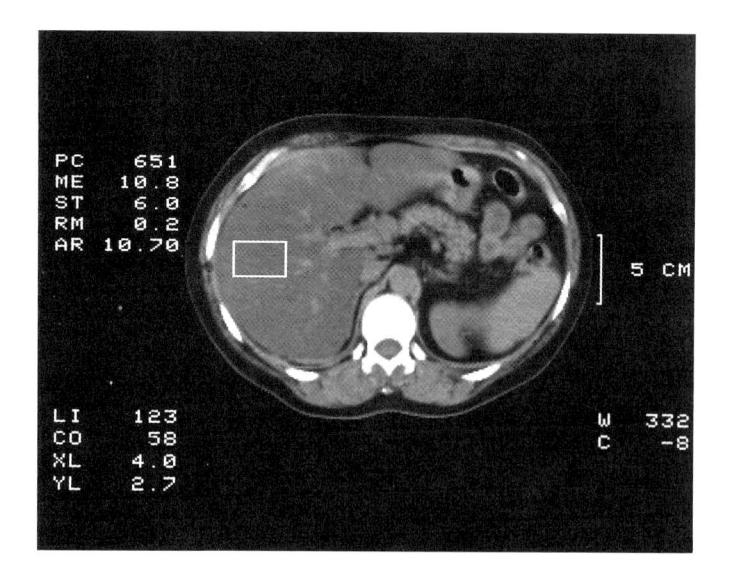

Fig. 3.11
In the simpest case, quantitative CT consists of determining the average of the CT values in a delineated area (ROI). In the example shown, an attempt was made to determine the fat content of the liver.

A very important reason for the often only limited acceptance of quantitative diagnoses is that it has never been possible to compare CT number values between different systems. It has been shown in CT publications that, for certain types of scanners, the CT number values are unreliable for quantitative diagnoses, because they depend upon the size and position of the patient within the gantry aperture [4, 5]. An awareness of such problems has only come about relatively recently.

Scattered radiation, beam hardening problems or a scanning field appreciably smaller than the gantry aperture are the principal reasons why CT number values for these scanners vary with the size and position of the patient (see 1.5). The SOMATOM concept offers the optimum design for eliminating or greatly reducing these effects. This is achieved through the utilization of a rotating detector, which effectively collimates against scattered radiation, flat copper filters to minimize beam hardening effects, and a large scanning field.

The particular strong point of SOMATOM relative to other CT systems can be easily demonstrated by comparative evaluation of the accuracy and the reproducibility of CT number values resulting from widely different scanning conditions. Use of the dual-energy method, at present undergoing testing (see 3.3.5), is expected to extend the possibilities of quantitative computed tomography substantially.

The quantitative assessment of a CT image as supplementary or even as the decisive diagnostic information is possible on a routine basis at any time, as long as suitable means of image evaluation are at hand.

3.2.3 Dynamic Computed Tomography

In the CT literature, the term "dynamic computed tomography" is used to describe all CT applications with the aim of obtaining information on the blood supply to and the function of an organ. This entails the rapid scanning sequence of a slice and the assessment of contrast medium behavior with time following its intravenous injection. ECG-gated cardiac scans and fast, automated scans of entire organs or sections of organs are also included in dynamic CT. According to the different clinical problems involved, the fields of application for dynamic computed tomography are variously described in the literature as Serio CT, Angio CT, Sequential CT, Cardio CT or Dynamic CT with automatic table advance (Auto CT).

Requirements for Dynamic Computed Tomography

The following requirements are essential for successful clinical application:
- ▷ fast scanning sequences
- ▷ possibility for quantitative evaluation
- ▷ high stability over time
- ▷ high contrast sensitivity
- ▷ flexibility of operation and reproducibility of scan parameters

A fast scanning sequence is an essential requirement for imaging rapidly occurring physiological processes. This demands short scanning times, high scanning rates and short deadtimes between scans. The most pronounced differentiation of lesions is usually possible during the influx phase of the contrast medium bolus, e. g. to image vascular changes (aneurysms, arteriovenous malformations) or to examine the arterial and capillary phases in parenchymal organs. Here, a large number of scans is necessary within a few seconds (Fig. 3.12).

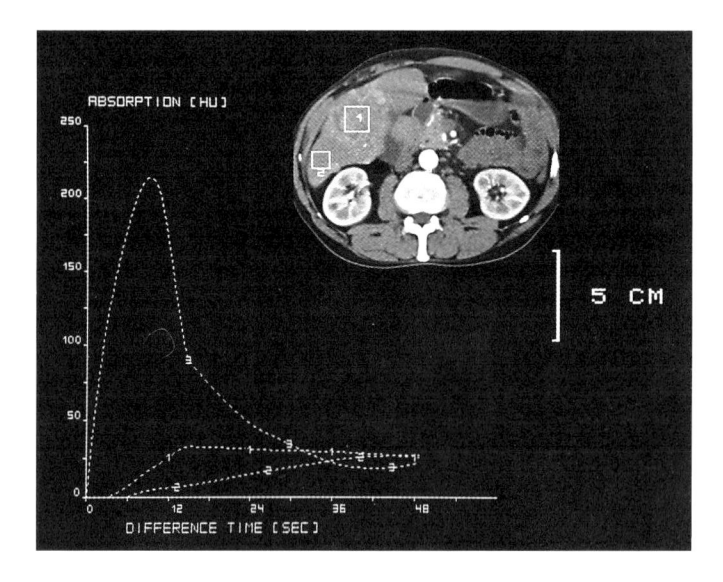

Fig. 3.12
With dynamic CT, following injection of the contrast medium bolus, a rapid sequence of scans (in this example, 12 scans per minute) is made of a slice. This determines the behavior of the contrast medium over a period of time. The method permits the recognition of different contrasts in regions 1 and 2, here seen only in the early phase.

In order to view an entire organ in a short time while the contrast medium concentration is high, a high scanning frequency and rapid table advance are again necessary (Fig. 3.13). For direct imaging of the heart during a phase of motion, scanning times on the order of magnitude of a fraction of a second are desirable. The most stringent requirements are thus very demanding, and they must be reconciled with the physical possibilities of the scanning system along with all additional requirements.

The possibility of quantitative evaluation, such as the numerical description of density variations in marked areas and their representation in graphic form, is important. The available software generally offers enough possibilities. The important point is that the quality of data suffices for such an analysis. The individual images from a dynamic series should be free of artifacts, and the scanning system should be capable of quantitative CT operation (see 3.2.2).

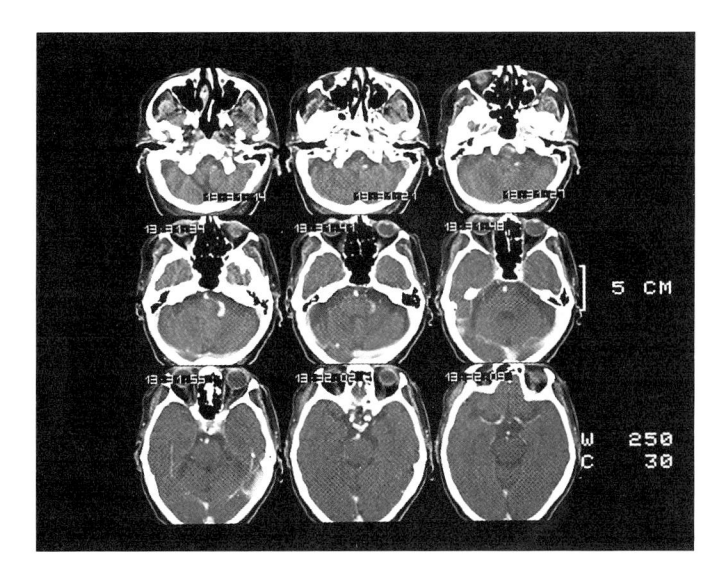

Fig. 3.13
In order to examine an entire organ as quickly as possible after the introduction of contrast medium, scanning and table advance can be preprogrammed for automatic execution (Auto CT). The nine scans shown were generated in 55 seconds.

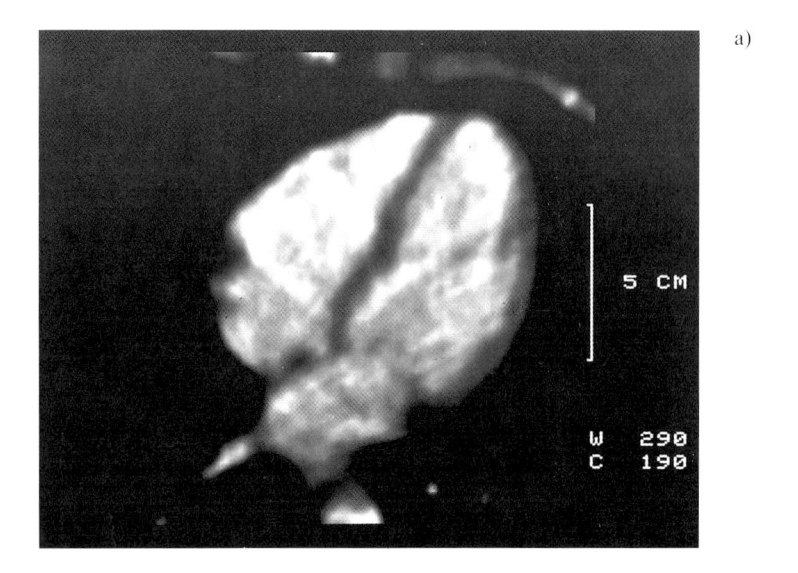

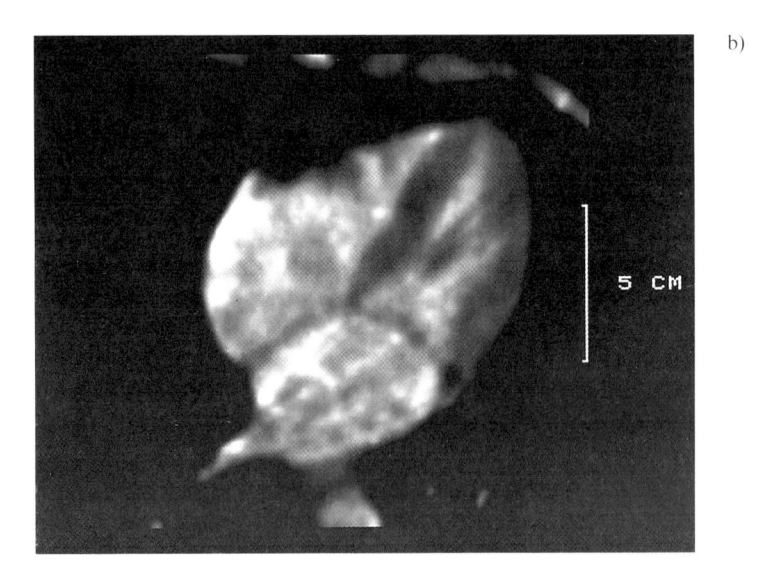

Fig. 3.14
Reconstruction of a cardiac slice in end diastole (a) and end systole (b), taken from eight ECG-gated CT scans

In addition, it is necessary that the scanner remain stable over a period of time, particularly for ECG-gated scans of the heart (Fig. 3.14). Here, the data from consecutive scans must be used to construct a single set of data, which is then used as the basis for reconstructing images of the heart in a phase of motion [6]. This procedure is then extremely sensitive to artifacts arising from fluctuations in the generator, X-ray tube or series of motions executed by the scanner. As a result, its implementation is only possible with scanning systems offering superior stability during the scanning procedure.

Another important requirement for quantitative evaluation is high contrast sensitivity. This is because, clinically, the documentation of very small changes in contrast medium enrichment in adjacent regions of an organ, and not the imaging of the bolus in the larger blood vessels, is of interest. This means that sufficiently high mAs values must be available for each scan in dynamic CT.

The requirement for greater flexibility of operation and greater reproducibility of the image results is largely a matter of system control and software. The important point here is the free selection of different scanning frequencies during a series, e.g. the possibility to preprogram the maximum scanning frequency in the early phase of the bolus input, followed by lower scanning frequencies, and then run the entire sequence automatically. This applies in a similar way to the automated, i.e. fastest possible, examination procedure for an entire organ or region of an organ (Auto CT).

Technical Followup Considerations

At this point, we wish to discuss the technical problems arising from the implementation of these requirements. For this, it is necessary to discuss the individual system components.

There are no insurmountable problems involving the detector system, scanning electronics and data acquisition. The effort for technical development is of course greater, and as a result the costs as well. This is true whether the scanning system has a rotating or a stationary detector system.

From the point of view of construction, there are no differences between these two systems in regard to attaining the shortest possible scanning times. In both cases, large masses (either the X-ray tube and detector or the X-ray tube along with the counterweights needed for rotational balance) must be accelerated over a short time, decelerated following scanning and then again accelerated in the opposite direction of rotation. The additional requirements of good image quality, extreme precision and stability in the scanning process must also be satisfied while these large masses are rotating.

The forces arising from the accelerations are however so large that the scanning frequencies of present-day systems cannot be increased very much further.

The limiting factor in regard to these requirements is nevertheless the X-ray tube. It is well known that every X-ray tube has a limited output. Extremely short scans are generally carried out with correspondingly low mAs values (see 3.1.3). The mAs value or equivalently the dose, which is proportional to this, then determines the contrast sensitivity (see 1.4). Depending upon the particular application, a certain contrast sensitivity and consequently a defined mAs value must be selected. This in turn also determines the maximum number of scans in a series for the given type of X-ray tube, depending above all on the heat loading capacity of the anode.

There is no point in further reducing the scanning time without being able to guarantee an adequate dose. This means that the X-ray tube is the limiting system component for dynamic CT.

The Possibilities of Present-day CT Technology

We have now defined the goals and problems. It is of paramount importance in system development for dynamic CT to aim for the greatest possible X-ray tube output and, logically then, for the greatest possible detector efficiency. The geometric efficiency and the quantum efficiency of the detector system are of course also of particular importance in connection with the patient dose. This consideration must be regarded very seriously in dynamic CT.

In order to describe the general considerations discussed concretely above in regard to how well these requirements are actually fulfilled and how well they could be fulfilled, we refer to the example of SOMATOM. In all areas of application for dynamic CT discussed, this scanning system offers special solutions (the parameters currently offered are found in the applicable data sheets).

Serio CT

The maximum scanning frequency is twelve scans per minute. Making use of a split image (reconstruction of three individual images separated in time from a single scan), a maximum rate of 36 images per minute is then possible. For frequencies up to nine scans per minute, the image appears instantaneously, as soon as the scan is finished, permitting continuous control of the contrast medium concentration and the slice being scanned. With the maximum scanning frequency, up to 25 scans can be performed without interruption.

With preprogramming, it is possible in a dynamic study to select up to five regions, each with a different scanning frequency.

Along with numerous diagnostic functions and models for the graphic representation of data, the evaluation software offers a CINE DISPLAY. This feature repeatedly displays twelve images at a speed which can be freely selected (up to 30 images/s). It allows assessing the contrast medium dynamics more satisfactorily than in terms of the commonly used parameter images.

Auto CT

Very fast scanning sequences with automatic slice advance are particularly interesting for the examination of a complete body region as quickly as possible, following a bolus injection. A maximum of 11 body scans or 7.5 head scans per minute is possible. With immediate image verification, these figures are 8.5 and 6.2 per minute, respectively. The CINE DISPLAY is also available here, allowing a spatial scanning of the region being examined.

Cardio CT

Only ECG-gated scanning techniques are of interest here, since they permit the reconstruction of blur-free images correlated with cardiac phase from several scans of a slice. Between six and twelve scans are taken of the same slice with immediate image verification.

Clinical experience has demonstrated clearly that the instantaneous image is indispensable for monitoring the contrast medium concentration and the respiration of the patient for cardiac studies. During the scan, the ECG data are automatically matched to the corresponding scanning data and stored in memory. The beginning of a scan is triggered by the ECG (prospective gating), giving the most effective method of data acquisition. A complete set of data is then synthesized for the cardiac phase selected from the individual scans and reconstructed as an image (Fig. 3.14). This procedure has been in clinical use since 1978 [7]. SOMATOM is the only scanner on the market offering this prospective gating capability.

3.2.4 Biopsy and Stereotaxis

Biopsies and stereotactic operating procedures can be performed with various aims and techniques. In regard to the requirements imposed on CT scanners, however, these all have much in common. This section considers only needle puncture biopsy methods. Under the guidance of radiological monitoring, the needle is introduced into a region to be explored or into a lesion already located and a tissue sample removed for histological studies. Computed tomography is a necessary part of this procedure when simpler methods, such as ultrasound or X-ray fluoroscopy, are unable to locate the region in question or the structures between the point of insertion and the target volume with sufficient accuracy. In difficult cases, the biopsy must be performed with the aid of a stereotactic frame (see above).

The use of CT with stereotactic operating procedures, usually therapeutic measures, is very similar. Here too, a volume of interest must be defined and the most satisfactory path to it determined. Depending upon the procedure, e.g. cutting out a small tumor or the implantation of radioactive seeds, the requirements may be more demanding than for a biopsy. During the examination, the patient is normally secured in a stereotactic frame, which defines a coordinate system. For simple programs, the coordinates are calculated for any given points in the CT image, in particular for the point of interest and the point of insertion, in this system and transmitted to a viewing device. According to the degree of difficulty, the surgical procedure can be performed either in the CT system, with or without immediate image verification, or in the operating room (Fig. 3.15).

The specific requirements imposed upon the CT scanner are determined by the specific dangers of the surgical procedure. The spatial resolution, which determines the accuracy for the locations of the point of interest and the needle, is particularly important. It is the slice thickness, and not the resolution in the image (which should be better than 1 mm as defined by the diameter of the smallest distinguishable bore holes in a resolution test: see 1.2), which determines the accuracy of position from the CT point of view. Still more important is, however, to be able to carry out the entire examination quickly: in particular, the image must appear as soon as the scan is finished. Since complications can never be ruled out altogether, the instantaneous image is a requirement of the utmost priority. Since a larger number of scans may be necessary for slices of 1 or 2 mm thickness, a high scanning frequency is also very desirable.

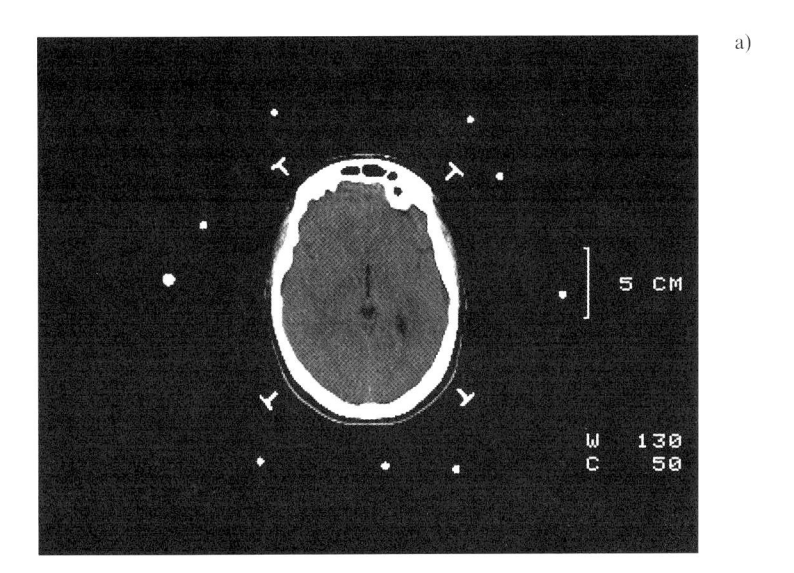

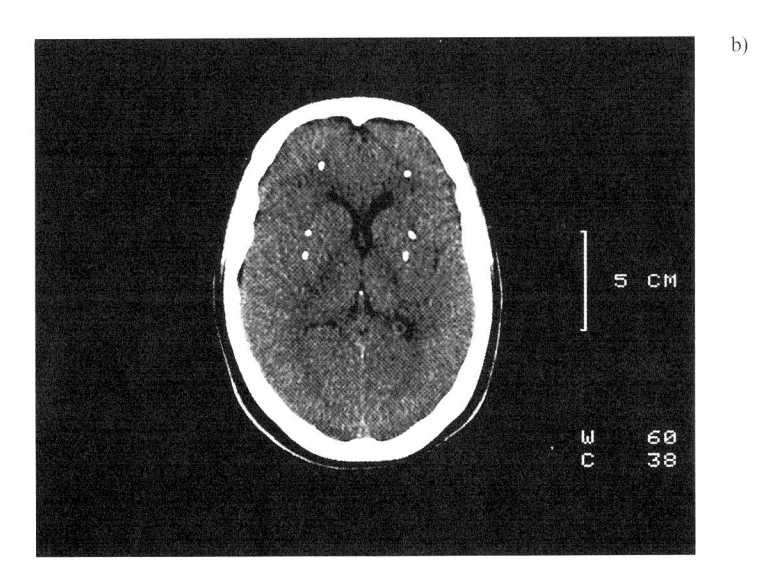

Fig. 3.15
Viewing coordinates can be calculated from scans showing the patient's skull with a stereotactic frame (a). The control scan (b) shows the correct electrode implantation.

3.2.5 Radiation Therapy Planning

Computed tomography has brought about enormous progress in the diagnosis of tumors and thus indirectly also an improved basis for therapeutic decisions. In addition, it directly provides information of importance for optimal radiation therapy planning. This does not immediately imply a special application of CT; a more accurate description would be a specialized extension to the processing of CT information. In any case, this does entail specific demands on the CT scanner itself, in particular on the interface to the therapy planning system (Fig. 3.16).

The most important information to be gained for therapy planning from a series of CT images consists of details on the size and volume of a lesion and its exact topographic-anatomic location in space relative to neighboring structures. In order to prescribe dose values, the total volume to be irradiated is needed. For a reliable calculation of the dose values, a reproducible and highly accurate matching of the local density values to the CT number values measured must be guaranteed. In other words, the same requirements must be imposed on a CT scanner as discussed above in connection with the possibilities of achieving a quantitative diagnosis.

The transfer of CT images to the therapy planning system used can be problematical when the system components are from different manufacturers, involving the use of different formats and computer components. It is certainly advantageous to have the therapy planning unit from the CT manufacturer.

This offers another advantage also. In the simplest case, it is possible to save on costs and space requirements by integrating the two systems. The SOMADOS system serves here as an example. With a planning system which is separate from the CT system, commonly found only in large therapy departments, the same hardware and software components can be used to advantage. A particularly striking example for this is the Siemens therapy planning system (SIDOS, EVADOS), which in its present version also takes advantage of the high speed computer developed especially for CT image reconstruction. A consideration of the expected trend in future developments for therapy planning systems suffices to make clear that, in regard to computer speed and accuracy, we are already approaching the limits inherent in the minicomputers generally used. The importance of having such an integrated system is therefore apparent.

The demand for high-speed computation results from the fact that the objects which influence the radiation field, such as blocks, mantel fields, compensators, etc., substantially increase the computation time for each stationary field.

The trend in computer-supported therapy planning is also clearly towards attaining a high level of accuracy. Only the use of complex computer methods and the continual refinement of the computer grid in order to attain more exact isodose generation permit reaching a greater level of accuracy. The minicomputer based radiation therapy planning systems attempting to satisfy these requirements are

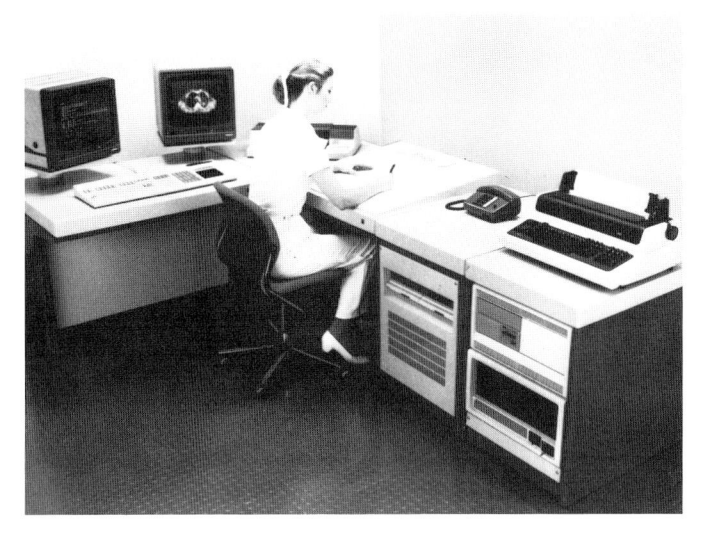

a) Therapy planning workstation

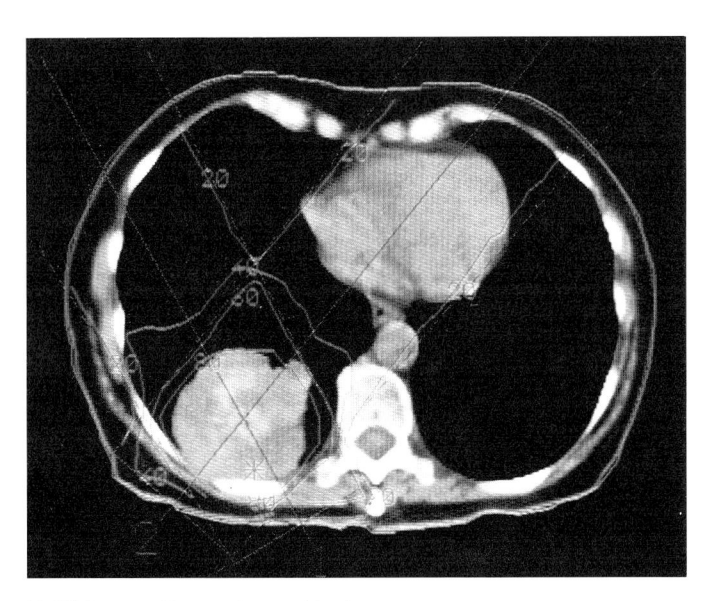

b) CT image with superimposed isodose curves

Fig. 3.16 Therapy planning

altogether inadequate, because the computation time needed is then intolerably long, especially for moving-beam therapy.

The use of an array processor offers an entirely satisfactory solution here. In the present case, a special version, BSP11-TP, of the processor used in the CT system reconstructs a stationary field having 14,000 points within 0.2 s. Details of the therapy planning system can be taken from other sources. The decisive considerations here are those pointing to the future. The true three-dimensional radiation therapy planning, based on a large number of CT slices, expected for the future will require a large working memory and extremely high speeds of computation. A processor having this capability is practically indispensable for the realization of such a system.

3.3 Medical Research

3.3.1 Problems and Goals of CT

Refinements in X-ray computed tomography, e. g. in image reconstruction algorithms and system technology – both of which have advanced to a high level of development –, have led to a shift in research activities toward emphasizing new CT applications. One result of this trend is that, increasingly, the impetus toward new developments in CT comes from the user. However, apart from basic clinical research, the user is limited by the design of his system. Research activities, such as developing new or improved clinical procedures, almost always imply the need for system characteristics above and beyond those offered for routine operation. It is not always possible for the manufacturer to provide this retrofit capability. One approach to solving this problem is to design the CT system to be as flexible as possible. This allows for the maximum possibility of implementing new applications without the need for complicated system modifications, which offers the advantage of wide-ranging control and monitoring of the system by means of the software. Exactly this has been done throughout the entire SOMATOM. This means advantages not only for the research applications discussed here, but also a concept aiming to provide the capability to respond to future demands.

The question then arises, which concrete requirements are most often advanced for research-oriented applications. The possibility of implementing the user's own formulations for the processing and evaluation of images is usually regarded as a very important condition for conducting independent research. Such work is made possible at all or made very much easier through direct access to the CT hardware (in particular to the image processor, image memory and such operating elements as light pens and potentiometers). It is not practicable or useful in routine operation to transfer CT images to any desired computer system or to modify or attempt to diagnose the images in the absence of visual control and subsequently transmit them back to the CT system. Another requirement often mentioned among users involved with basic research in computed tomography is direct access to the primary scan data used to reconstruct the images.

Siemens has frequently offered such possibilities to users of SOMATOM in the course of their research activities. There are program libraries available which enable every user to access the CT hardware. This will be discussed below in greater detail in the context of examples for research projects in computed tomography.

A complete list of all conceivable clinical research applications requiring system modifications in regard to scanning techniques, image reconstruction, image postprocessing or image evaluation would be very extensive. Especially for the postprocessing, manipulation or evaluation of CT images, there is practically no limit to the degree of refinement or complexity. This is particularly true when automatic contour recognition, pattern recognition or structure analysis also come into play, since there are numerous approaches to these problems throughout the CT literature. In each such case, as well as for the examples discussed below, the validity of the method of evaluation or the value of the method must first be demonstrated. The manufacturer can only make the apparatus available; it is left to the researcher to answer these questions.

3.3.2 Example: Evaluation of CT Cardiac Images

The evaluation of cardiac radiographs according to geometrical models to determine volumes and the resulting functional parameters, such as the ejection fraction, represents a long-standing problem. For a long time, X-ray films were manually evaluated according to a variety of methods with these determinations in mind [8].

It is of immediate interest to apply such methods of evaluation to ECG-gated CT scans of the heart (see 3.2.3).

Furthermore, it is interesting that a CT image additionally allows the quantitative regional diagnosis of the heart muscle and its ability to contract. Since a computer-based evaluation can be made very quickly, several diagnostic models can be tested and their usefulness compared.

With such an analysis in mind, one user has written a system of programs in FORTRAN, which runs on the CT system and on the separate diagnostic console. The programs call upon the user library (USRLIB), so that light pens, potentiometers and all graphics possibilities are available. The comfort of operation and the program running time are thus similar to those for the system programs. The user-developed program must only run separately from the system programs.

The diagnosis of cardiac images, previously scanned with heart-phase correlation and then reconstructed, runs according to the following steps: the end-diastolic image is read into image memory and appears on the monitor. With the aid of the light pen, the base and contour of the ventricle are determined point by point. Every input can be erased. In the following step, the program requests selection of the connecting line between the center of the base and the point farthest away on the ventricular contour as the longitudinal axis of the ventricle. A potentiometer permits the continuous shifting of the axis end points in order to achieve a better orientation of the longitudinal axis. The determination of the transverse axes and the thickness of the heart muscle follow a similar procedure. The program first draws in the lines determined by the programs, following which the operator can try out different lines. As soon as all inputs have been entered (Fig. 3.17a), the program calculates the thicknesses of the heart muscle, the lengths of the axes and the total and regional ventricle surfaces in true scale. The volume is calculated using different formulas according to the surface-length method, surface-cross section method, summation slice method and models incorporating the user's own modification.

The end-systolic image (Fig. 3.17b), as well as any number of images of the cardiac cycle following, is taken from the same scan. Along with the systolic values, the percent change between systole and diastole and the stroke volume are calculated also. The operator can output these results onto the printer or the monitor screens in any form desired; it is even possible to photographically copy them directly in slide format (Fig. 3.17b).

The entire diagnosis requires less than two minutes. Along with saving time and increasing accuracy by comparison with the manual evaluation of films, it is especially important for the operator that his own formulations are taken into account as he wishes.

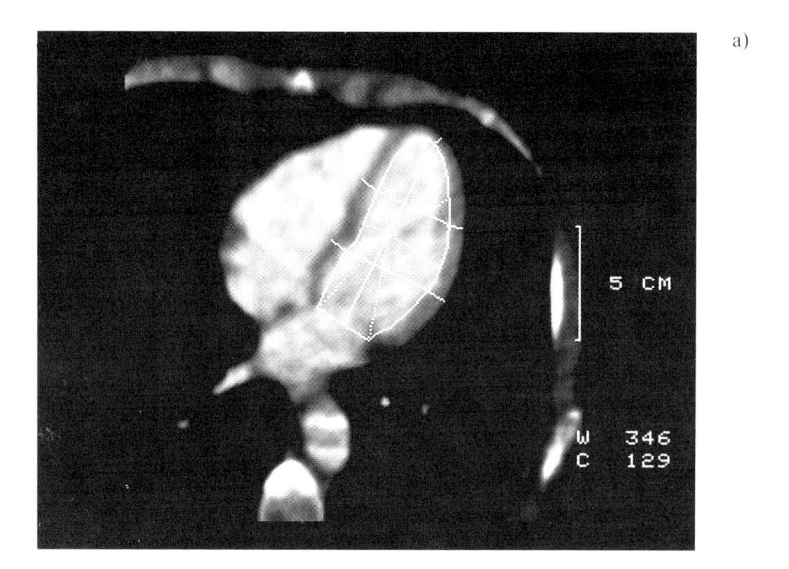

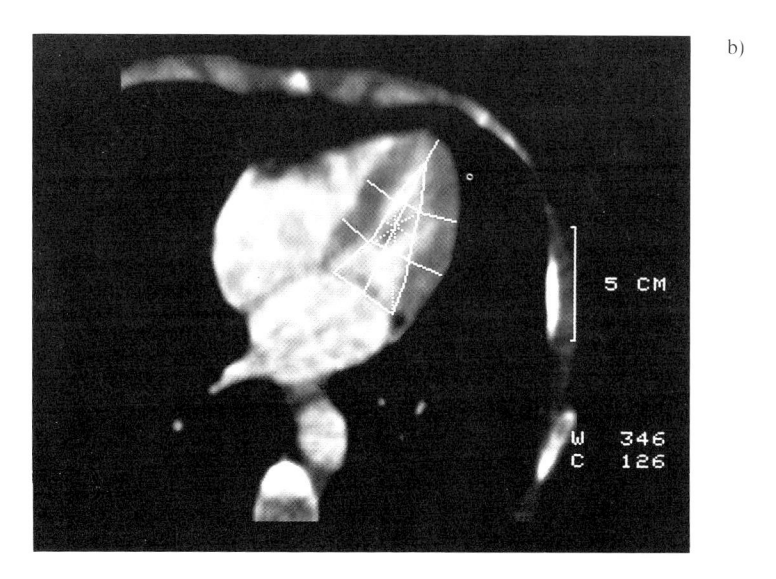

Fig. 3.17
Evaluation of CT cardiac images with user programs: the contour is inputted to the diastolic (a) and systolic (b) image using a light pen. The axes are taken from the program, but can be modified at will by the operator. Further evaluation of the images, up to and including reconstruction and outputting the results (c), takes less than two minutes with this program.

c)

	DIAST.	SYST.	(D-S)/D
10.2.24			17-APR-80
EV.-C.	100 %	0 %	
MYOC. AB	0.8	1.5	86. %
MYOC. CD	0.8	1.6	114. %
F.-C.	0.4	1.1	178. %
L	8.8	6.3	28. %
Q1	3.9	1.9	51. %
Q2	3.5	1.1	68. %
Q0	3.7	1.5	59. %
F	28.7	10.0	65. %
RF1	2.6	0.5	80. %
RF2	1.3	0.2	82. %
RF3	8.0	2.0	76. %
RF4	4.1	0.5	87. %
RF5	6.8	1.8	74. %
VFLM	79.4	13.4	83. %
VFQM	55.4	7.9	86. %
VQM	62.6	7.6	88. %
VSSM	76.4	15.3	80. %
SVFLM			66.1
SVFQM			47.5
SVQM			55.0
SVSSM			61.1

Fig. 3.17 (continued)

3.3.3 Example: Topogram as a Diagnostic Aid

Digital survey scans to help in selecting the CT slice planes or as a basis for their documentation (Figs. 3.3, 3.6, 3.7) are now widely used. We mention in passing that the basis of this technique, used with different types of scanners having varying image quality (see 2.2.5), derives from our own patent (German patent no. 2613809, U.S. patent no. 4174481).

The technical scanning parameters and with these also the image quality have improved considerably with time. In particular, the flexibility in the selection of different scanning field sizes, mAs values and directions of projection has increased. In regard to the development of digital radiography, which has taken place parallel to this, the question also arises of necessity to what extent this scanning mode can be of direct assistance for diagnoses and what form of image reconstruction or postprocessing is most useful.

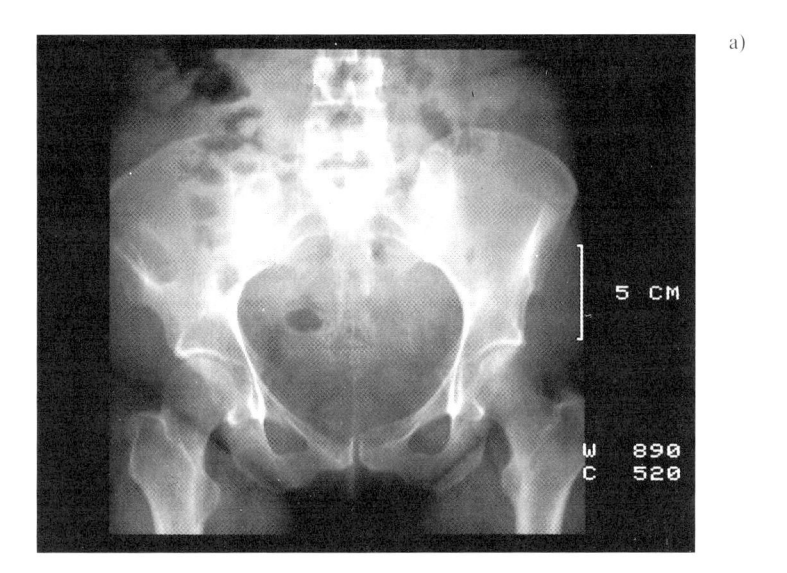

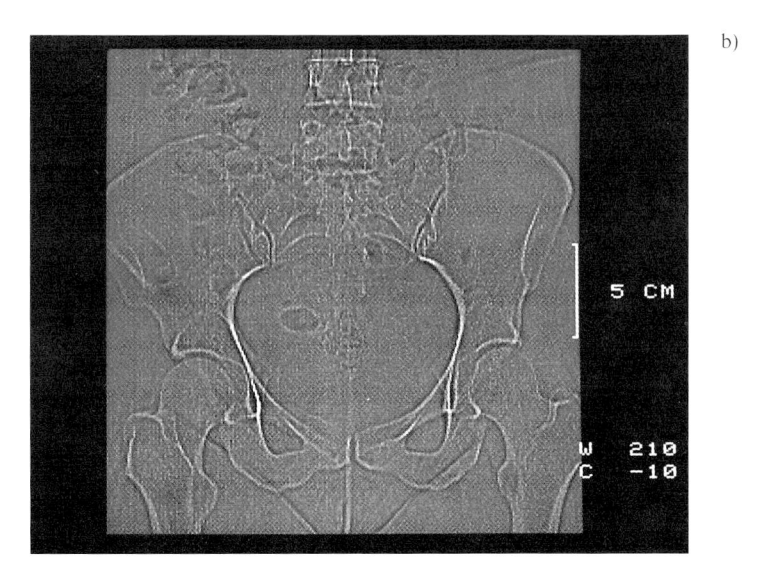

Fig. 3.18
Digital image processing offers the means to modify the image characteristics of a scan over a wide range: (a) original image, (b) "contour image", (c) image processed through a high-pass filter, (d) enlargement of a section from c

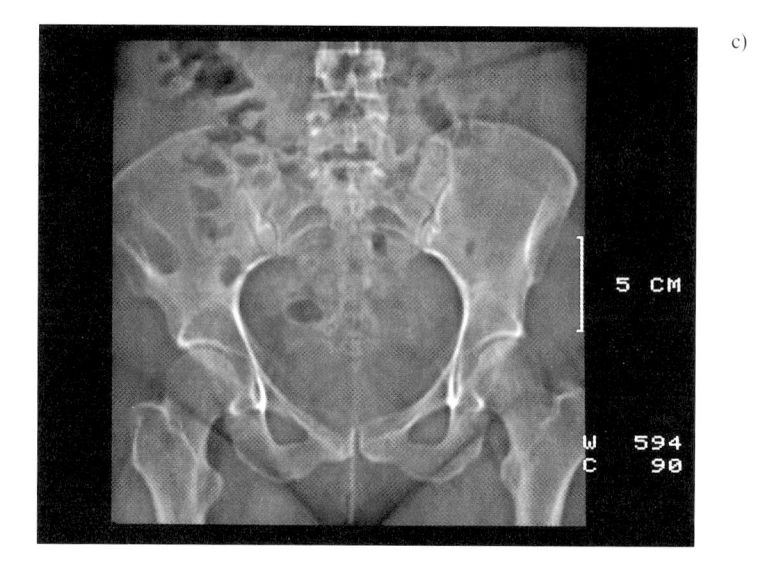

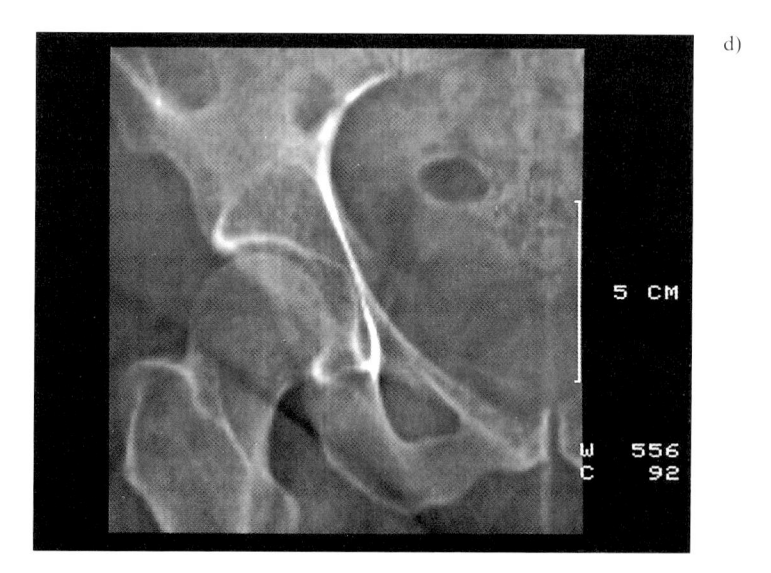

Fig. 3.18 (continued)

The goal is the selection of image characteristics which best allow the uniform recognition of details throughout the entire image. For example, in scans of the thorax, the lung region should be as easy to diagnose as the mediastinal region, and at the same time the contrast level should be kept as high as possible. The aim therefore is to take full advantage of both the broad dynamic range and the high level of contrast sensitivity offered by the digital system.

As demonstrated in Figures 3.18 a to d, digital image processing offers a number of possibilities [9]. The difficulty is in optimizing these for clinical applications.

Several medical institutes have dealt with this problem using SOMATOM systems and in doing so implemented their own algorithms. One necessary condition was the accessibility of scanning data. Here, scanning data refers to the scan values actually registered at each detector element and then preprocessed. Image data are then derived from these, i.e. images are reconstructed. Initial attempts to process images on a normal computer without regard to the CT system used led to programs requiring several hours for each reconstruction.

The problem was solved by using a high-speed CT processor. It was achieved in cooperation with SOMATOM users through the CT development laboratory, where program libraries for accessing the image processing computer in FORTRAN are now available. This reduced the computation time for each image to 20 seconds.

With these high-speed programs, it was possible to try out a large number of different reconstruction parameters and filters under clinical conditions. The results indicated that, for different clinical applications, different filters and reconstruction parameters should be available. This was taken into consideration in the system software for SOMATOM. In the meantime, it has been amply demonstrated that the topogram, particularly with optimized image reconstruction, can serve as the primary criterion for diagnosis in some clinical applications and, by way of direct comparison with conventional film-screen systems, shows definite advantages [10].

3.3.4 Example: Chronogram

The chronogram represents a special, rapid scanning modality offered by SOMATOM. It is used only for determining the contrast medium concentration curves. During scanning, the X-ray tube, detector and patient all remain stationary. A pulsed beam, e.g. 256 pulses in regular intervals of 100 ms, is applied and its attenuation measured repeatedly in the slice selected. After subtracting the time-independent background, the behavior of the contrast medium concentration can be represented with high temporal resolution.

This principle is similar to that forming the basis of digital subtraction angiography. However, the chronogram is limited to only one CT slice and does not image an entire organ (Fig. 3.19a).

A number of medical institutes have shown interest in this scanning modality. In order for the user to be able to evaluate the scans as he wishes, the scanning data must be made available. Diagnostic programs were constructed independently of the system software by making use of the program library (USRLIB). The first processing steps consist of background subtraction and the selection and representation of bolus curves (Fig. 3.19a).

One of the first projects involving the chronogram was designed to determine accurately and quantitatively the influence of various injection parameters, such as speed, volume and location of injection, on the bolus form and the enhancement which can be expected for it. This requires only the determination of peak time, height and FWHM value of the curve, easily determined interactively or with the user's own program [11].

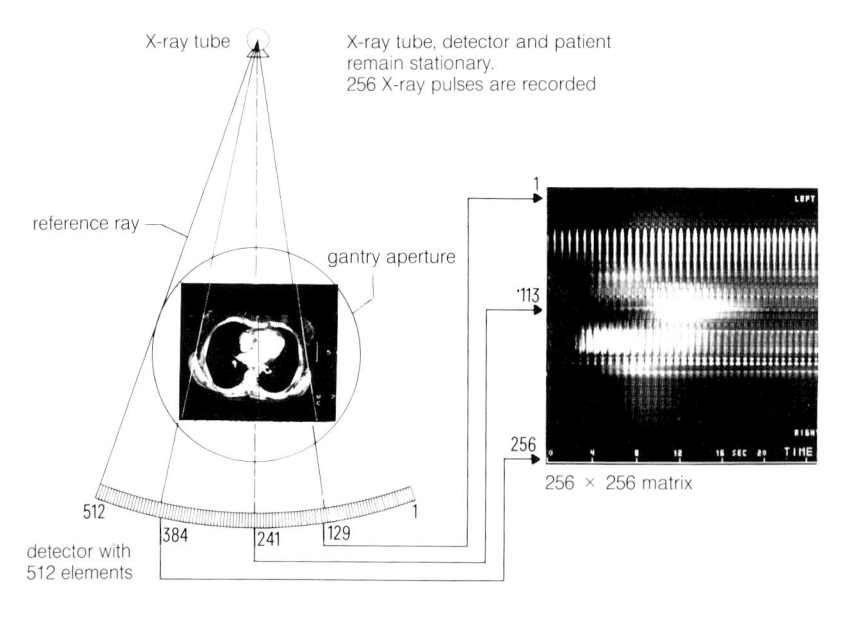

Fig. 3.19a
Scanning principle and image representation for chronogram scans. Changes in the beam attenuation following the introduction of contrast medium are measured with a high level of temporal resolution and plotted column-wise as a function of time.

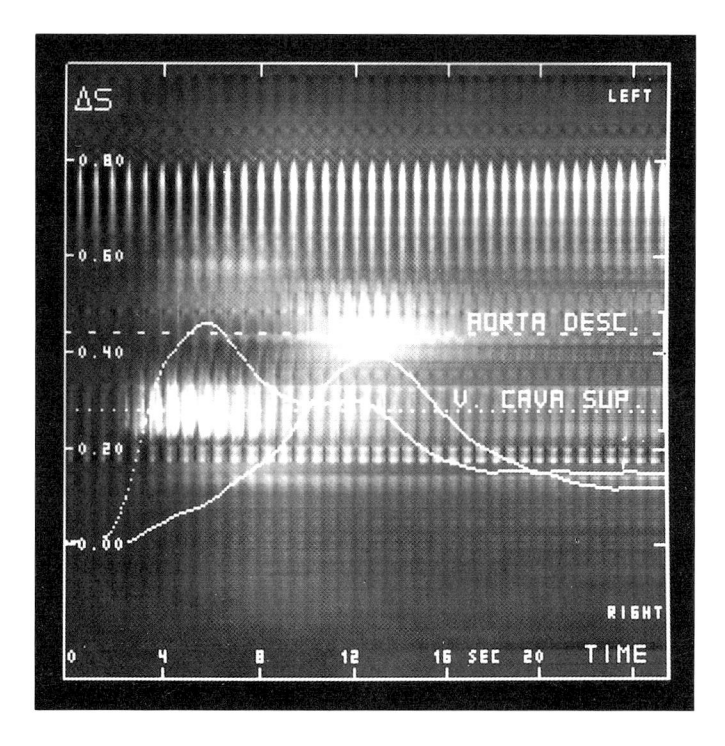

Fig. 3.19b
The contrast medium concentration curves can be plotted for any blood vessel and used for the quantitative determination of blood flow values

In another project, blood flow values were determined quantitatively for the brain from chronogram-bolus curves taken from near the base of the skull, using a modified transit time method [12]. The user was able to link together FORTRAN programs already available from applications in nuclear medicine for curve plotting and evaluation programs. The programs permit the rapid, interactive (using light pen and potentiometer) selection of regions in the chronogram image for which the contrast medium concentration-time curves are to be plotted. They also evaluate the plots and display the results on the monitor screen.

3.3.5 Example: Dual-energy Method

CT images represent images of the linear attenuation coefficients for the volume elements of the slice imaged. They are therefore in no sense density images, as is often said incorrectly. The linear attenuation coefficient is a product of the material's attenuation characteristics for the X-ray beam employed and the local density. A number of relevant clinical problems result from this. If, for example, a node in the lung is represented in the CT image by increased values, it cannot be said with certainty if this is due to a diffuse calcification, i.e. to contributions from elements of higher atomic number, or to a fibrosis, i.e. an increase in density.

Scanning a slice with two different X-ray spectra permits calculating the density distribution of specific materials (Fig. 3.20) and displaying these as images along with the usual CT images. Electron density images based on these results and of value for radiation therapy planning can be displayed, as well as so-called "mononergetic" CT images. Their advantage is the elimination of the artifacts present in a conventional CT image due to spectral hardening.

Initial attempts to employ the dual-energy method in computed tomography followed shortly after its introduction in clinical practice [13, 14]. Even though its main advantages could be demonstrated clearly, the method has not gained wide acceptance in clinics. Due to the need for two scans separated in time by ten seconds or more and taken at two different values of high voltage, the method has proved to be too susceptible to patient movements. Even the slightest motion is enough to invalidate the evaluation of the data. Another problem is that the reference scanning data needed as the basis of an evaluation are generally not available to interested users from CT manufacturers.

The subject of the dual-energy methods has nevertheless been taken up again under more favorable conditions for SOMATOM systems. In order to minimize the effect of patient movements, auxiliary electronics was developed to permit switching between the two high-voltage values in millisecond intervals, i.e. from pulse to pulse, and obtaining the data for both voltages in a single scan. This advance has already proven of value in clinical practice. The modification of the scanning principle was possible, because a pulsed beam and not a continuous beam had always been used for SOMATOM (see 2.4). Moreover, the entire system proved to be flexible enough to allow introducing this new scanning mode into the already existing system.

The problem of accessing the scanning data no longer arises. In order to provide for the conduct of research by individual users interested in investigating and improving the dual-energy method, the scanning data were made available along with other important information within the system. This permits those institutions concerned with specialized research problems, in particular the representation of density for specific materials, to test their own methods of evaluation and postprocessing with the same system.

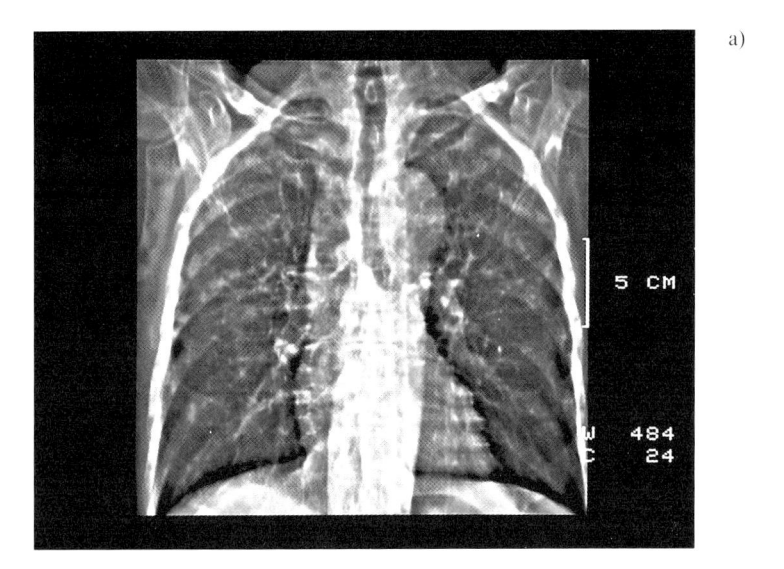

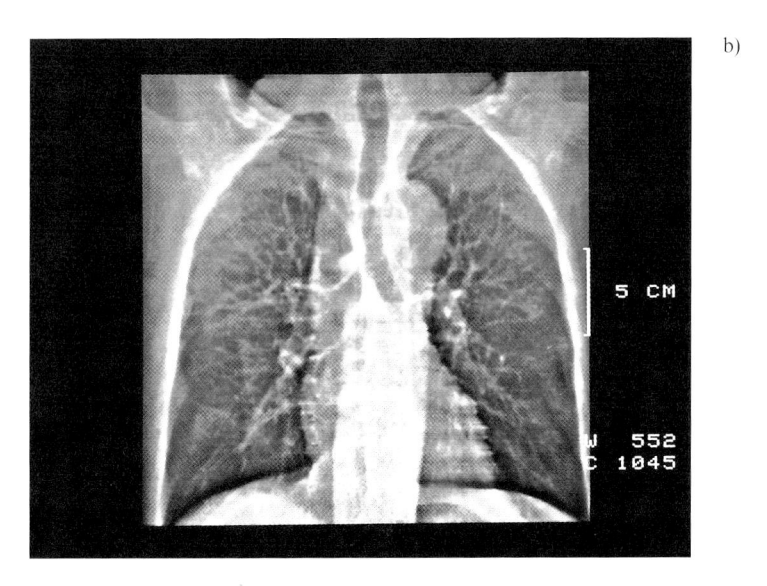

Fig. 3.20
Dual-energy topogram of a patient with metastases resulting from an oesophagus carcinoma. The standard scan (a) raises suspicion of pulmonary metastases. The material-selective reconstructions taken from scans with the dual-energy mode show unequivocally that an osteal process is the underlying problem. The "soft-tissue image" (b) is not cause for undue alarm, while the "bone image" (c) shows the presence of diffuse osteolysis.

c)

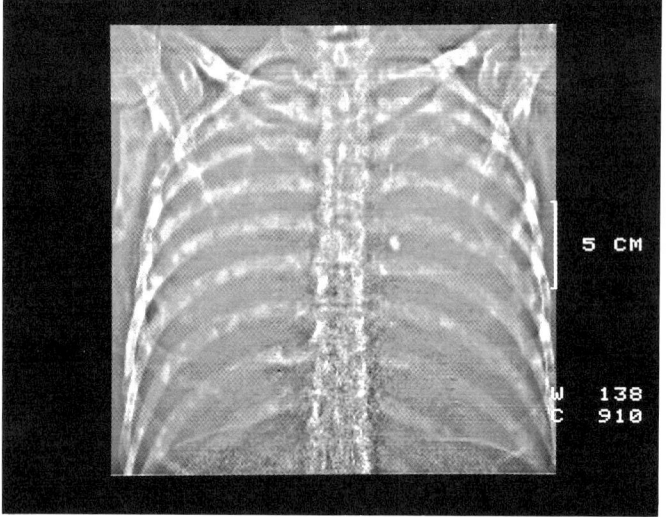

Fig. 3.20 (continued)

3.3.6 Conclusions

These few examples suffice to make the essential requirements for medical research using a CT system clear. Let us now summarize them in relation to system components, scanning method, image reconstruction, image postprocessing and diagnosis.

Modifications to the scanning method almost always lead to a critical situation, especially when the construction, system control or X-ray generation is affected, because the safety of the patient and an examination procedure free of disturbances must be guaranteed at all times. This means that such modifications can only be carried out by the manufacturer. Not all ideas are technically possible or physically justified.

Flexibility and room for modifications are the direct result of software control over the entire system. This concept allows modifications to the scanning method without the need to perform hardware modifications. In this regard, the pulsed beam has also proven itself.

For reasons of time and effort, the image reconstruction should always run on the CT system. Although the underlying data corrections and reconstruction algorithms are very complex, a few users have made their own contributions or pursued their own alternatives. A necessary condition for being able to do this was the possibility to access scanning data and related information from the manufacturer.

Image postprocessing and evaluation most frequently concern medical research employing CT systems with modified parameters. The list of examples is as long as the list of individual approaches to clinical problems or the number of possibilities of evaluating the data resulting from them. This applies just as well to individual documentation systems or quality control programs, such as checking out new models, e.g. for the evaluation of dynamic CT series, statistical analyses of tissue characterization or the determination of geometric parameters for orthopedic examinations.

The requirements are all nearly the same: the researcher wishes to access the image data from his own program, in order to investigate an individual or an innovative approach. After reconstructing the image, he wishes to process the data in real time and enter additional information freely into the image. In addition the results, graphs etc. should be displayed on the monitor screen. These requirements can generally be satisfied. The program library (USRLIB) includes modules which directly address the hardware and which can be called up by user-developed programs. The library programs have demonstrated their usefulness and reliability at a large number of institutions.

Literature

[1] Cann, C. E.; Genant, H. K.: Precise measurement of vertebral mineral content using computed tomography. J. Comput. Assist. Tomogr. 4, pp. 493–500, 1980
[2] Schmitt, W. G. H.; Hübner, K.-H.: Dichtebestimmungen normaler und pathologisch veränderter Lebergewebe als Basisuntersuchung zur computertomographischen Densitometrie von Fettlebern. Fortschr. Röntgenstr. 129, pp. 555–559, 1978
[3] Siegelman, S. S.; Zerhouni, E. A.; Leo, F. P.; Khouri, N. F.; Stitik, E. P.: CT of the solitary pulmonary nodule. Amer. J. Roentgenol. 135, pp. 1–13, 1980
[4] Levi, C.; Gray, J. E.; McCullough, E. C.; Hattery, R. R.: The unreliability of CT numbers as absolute values. Amer. J. Roentgenol. 139, pp. 443–447, 1982
[5] Hemmingson, A.; Jung, B.; Ytterbergh, C: Ellipsoidal body phantom for evaluation of CT scanners. J. Comput. Assist. Tomogr. 7, pp. 503–508, 1983
[6] Rogalsky, W.; Hahn, R.: Kardioaufnahmetechnik mit dem SOMATOM. Electromedica 50, pp. 51–55, 1982
[7] Lackner, K.; Thurn, P.: Computed tomography of the heart: ECG-gated and continuous scans. Radiology 140, pp. 413–420, 1981
[8] Lichtlen, P. R.: Koronarangiographie. Perimed-Verlag, Erlangen, 1979
[9] Kalender, W. A.; Hübener, K.-H.; Jass, W.: Optimization of Image Characteristics in Digital Scanned Projection Radiography. Radiology 149, pp. 299–303, 1983
[10] Hübener, K. H.: Scanned Projection Radiography of the Chest versus Standard X-ray Film: A Comparison of 250 Cases. Radiology 148, pp. 363–368, 1983
[11] Claussen, C. D.; Banzer, D.; Pfretzschner, C.; Kalender, W. A.; Schörner, W.: Bolus Geometry and Dynamics after Intravenous Contrast Medium Injection. Radiology 153, pp. 365–368, 1984
[12] Lindner, P.; Wolf, E.; Schad, N.: Assessment of Regional Blood Flow by Intravenous Injection of 99m-Technetium-Pertechnetate. Eur. J. Nucl. Med. 5, pp. 229–235, 1980
[13] Alvarez, R. E.; Macovski, A.: Energy-selective Reconstructions in X-ray Computerized Tomography. Phys. Med. Biol. 21, pp. 733–744, 1976
[14] Rutherford, R. A.; Pullan, B. R.; Isherwood, J.: Measurement of Effective Atomic Number and Electron Density Using an EMI Scanner. Neuroradiology 11, pp. 15–21, 1976

4 Cost-effectiveness of CT Systems

An intelligent discussion of cost-effectiveness for computed tomography must take into account the influence of this examination technique on other diagnostic methods, on the one hand, and the most effective utilization of the CT system itself, on the other hand. Concerning the influence of CT on diagnostic procedures commonly used previously, it is of course only possible to comment very generally, since this depends very much on the operating structure of the given hospital.

A study in the USA[1]) on the influence of computed tomography on other diagnostic procedures for head studies shows:

Percent cost savings using CT in head studies (based on 130 CT installations)

Radiography	20%
Angiography	20%
Pneumoencephalography	80%
Nuclear medicine	60%

The average cost savings amount to about 40%. As a second example, we refer to a study carried out in the Federal Republic of Germany. Equipping a clinic[2]) with one CT scanner each for whole-body and head region examinations over a period of four years led to the following reductions in the number of diagnoses made by other methods:

Angiography	30%
Pneumoencephalography	80%
Nuclear medicine	55%

Furthermore, in the field of neurosurgery a reduction of 16% in the length of hospital stay was achieved at the same time.

Efficient utilization of the CT scanner itself depends largely on the number of examinations that can be performed daily, which is determined in turn by the design concept and standard of quality of the scanner.

---

[1]) Mallinkrodt Institute of Radiology
[2]) Klinikum Mannheim, Neurochirurgie

4.1 Amortization and Number of Examinations

A comparison of acquisition costs, operating costs and income from diagnoses gives a simplified account of cost effectiveness.

Typical acquisition costs are:

    equipment (including options)
    transport and insurance
    construction, including radiation shielding, air conditioning, assembly and functional checkout

Operating costs include:

fixed costs	variable costs
rent, insurance	power consumption
service	archiving methods
financing	X-ray tube
training	consumable material

Personnel costs must also be considered. As with fixed operating costs, these are basically independent of the number of examinations performed. When a certain threshold level is exceeded, however, these costs rise abruptly, for example when an additional shift is initiated. Figure 4.1 illustrates such a cost-effectiveness analysis.

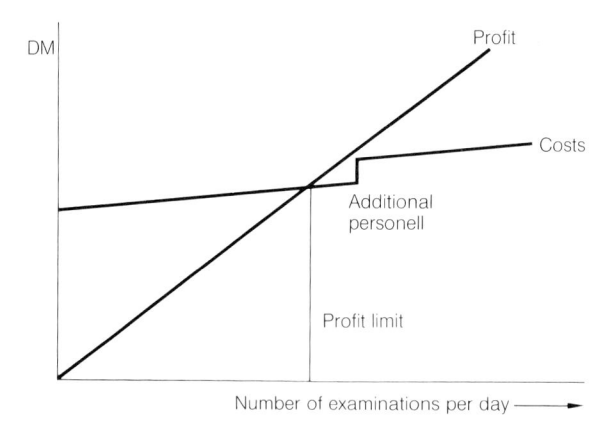

Fig. 4.1
Typical cost-benefit analysis for a CT system. Investment costs are high, while total costs yield a relatively flat profile. An abrupt cost increase occurs when an additional shift is initiated.

Characteristic of CT systems is the high initial outlay caused by the cost of acquisition, whereas the rise resulting from variable costs is relatively flat. This leads us to the conclusion that the number of examinations performed per day is decisive for cost-effective operation. The level of technical excellence of the CT system and an efficiently organized staff determine largely whether the CT system is amortized within the time expected.

For a modern CT scanner, such as SOMATOM, at least 15 patients can be examined comfortably during an 8 hour day. This requires at least one experienced X-ray technician full time and also the occasional presence of the responsible roentgenologist. Assuming that, on the average, each examination consists of 20 slices, then 300 scans are performed daily, along with the image reconstruction, archiving and documentation also entailed. This does not take into account the time for preparing and positioning the patient, which amounts to about 10 minutes per patient. As a rule, some of these procedures must be repeated several times for each examination, so that an exact analysis of where best to reduce the time required is of value (Fig. 4.2). We must then conclude that only about 1 minute is available for studying one slice, including diagnosis and documentation of the findings.

The rapid reconstruction of images and the largely automated scanning sequences are therefore decisive factors in the cost-effective operation of a CT scanner. The examination time can be greatly reduced only when instant display of the image is possible. Waiting between scanning and image reconstruction would mean that, following the examination of a sensitive region, the examination could not be ended immediately. This also means that there would be no possibility to immediately extend the CT study if so dictated by unexpected findings.

In order to avoid these disadvantages, such as are found with many CT systems, SOMATOM offers instantaneous image reconstruction. This also permits limiting the archiving and documentation to images relevant for diagnosis and makes optimum use of both storage media and X-ray film. Using a magazine camera controlled by the CT scanner, it is also possible to automate the documentation onto film, taking over still another task from the operating personnel.

It is equally as important for cost-effective operation that patient table time be kept to a minimum. The large scanning field for SOMATOM allows whole-body scanning, for example, without time-consuming patient positioning. The wide range of adjustment for the patient table greatly simplifies repositioning a patient and reduces the preparation time for patients in trauma or patients difficult to move. A mobile system for repositioning and transporting the patient prevents a bottleneck in the examination room due to time-consuming preparation of patients.

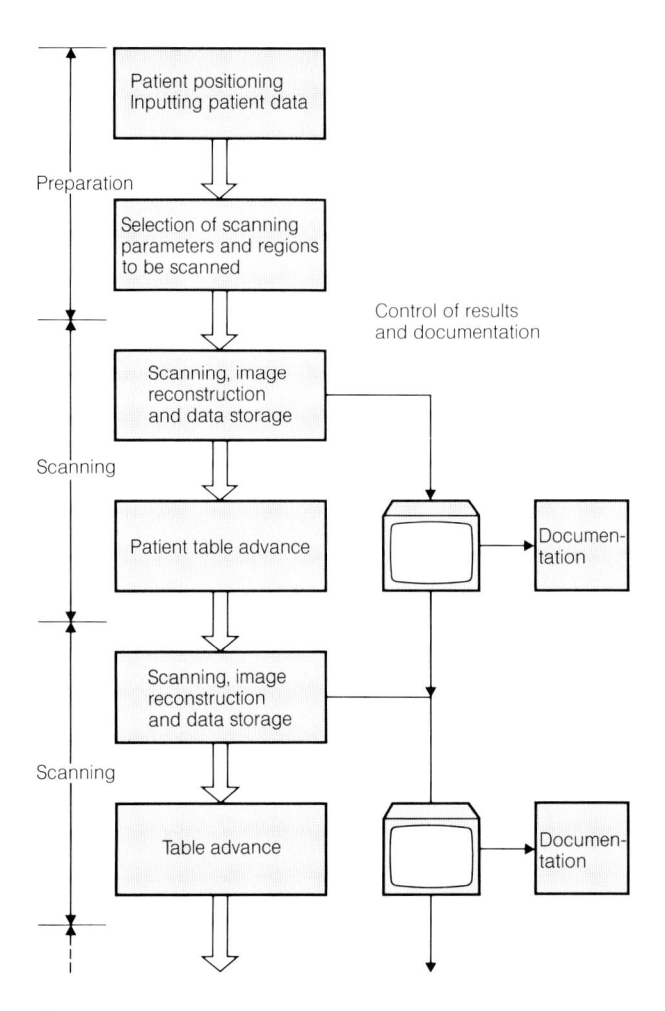

Fig. 4.2
CT scan sequence. The scanning, computation, display and documentation steps are performed repeatedly. The rapid execution of these steps greatly shortens the time of an examination.

Practice-oriented Considerations in Operating a CT Scanner

A high rate of patient throughput is only possible if a scanner is easy to operate. The following three requirements typify the needs of routine CT scanner operation:

▷ the patients should be examined during normal working hours, if possible

▷ the patient should only leave the examination room when the physician responsible has examined all findings

▷ the possibility of inserting unforeseen and emergency examinations with a minimum of disturbance to the routine examination plan

This means that, in addition to the instantaneous image reconstruction, quick scanning sequence and simplicity of patient positioning already mentioned, all operating sequences are also simple and time saving. The utilization of all possibilities inherent in a CT scanner in clinical practice takes for granted that all operating procedures are simple and easy to follow. The attention of physicians and medical personnel required to conduct an examination should not be unduly diverted by complicated computer dialog. A monitor-guided scanning procedure avoids erroneous settings, saves time and permits concentrating on the patient and the findings. SOMATOM, for example, making use of its built-in computer, has the most frequently needed operating commands and sequences preprogrammed: these can be called up by pressing the appropriate key.

This allows particularly simple operation in daily routine, as well as for emergencies. Even relatively inexperienced personnel can thus operate the system quickly and reliably under emergency conditions. All possibilities for the comprehensive evaluation of images or for medical research are still available without the need to burden routine operators with seldom-used functions. The entire system is designed so that clinical personnel can learn to position a patient on the table and document the results of an examination as easily as for other diagnostic equipment after only a relatively short period of training.

It is even possible to further improve the effectiveness of a CT system through the addition of a diagnostic console. This arrangement allows nearly continuous scanning with a minimum of time for assessing findings. A more exact image analysis and the use of additional diagnostic functions are also possible by means of a separate console. For a well designed system, routine operation from the scanner is largely unaffected by the diagnostic console, although this second console has access to all current information, including the completely new reconstruction of images.

Diagnostic Value of CT Images

Short examination times permit particularly cost-effective utilization of the CT system. At the same time, though, the results must also permit an unequivocal diagnosis. The evaluation criteria presented in the introductory chapters provide us with objective means for assessing image quality. The most important consideration is that the computed tomographic image (as a quantitative procedure for the determination of minute differences in attenuation) clearly reproduces these differences. Therefore, no appreciable variation in the attenuation values, usually given in Hounsfield units, can be tolerated over the entire scanning field. The resulting image will then be independent of the object position in the scanning field, an essential condition for the reproducibility of images. The same applies to the stability of CT values over a longer period of time, which must be monitored over a period of up to several months. A computed tomography system which cannot fulfil these requirements can only produce CT images for which a quantitative diagnosis is not possible.

Artifacts of physical-technical origin, such as partial-volume effects or streaks projecting from the end of a bone, can seriously detract from the CT image. SOMATOM offers the possibility to correct for these disturbances after viewing the initial image.

The sharpness of the image can be improved further if the image is reconstructed from a 512 x 512 matrix, which in effect requires no more time than the more frequently used 256 x 256 matrix. In order to take particularly cost-effective advantage of the magnetic memory, normal archiving can still be performed with a 256 x 256 matrix.

Reliability of a CT System

The reliability of a CT system is especially important in routine operation. In most radiological departments, there is only one CT system, so that a breakdown means the interruption or even termination of all CT examinations and evaluations. Since there are usually waiting lists for the patients to be examined, this would make a complete rearrangement of the scheduling necessary. It would also require that outpatients who could not undergo examinations as scheduled be asked to return at a later date.

A good indication of reliability is the quality of the X-ray tube used. The loading of the X-ray tube in computed tomography is about twice that of cineangiography, in addition to which about twice as many patients are examined daily with a CT scanner as with cine-angiography. If X-ray tubes having an inadequate life are used, this will unavoidably lead to a technical breakdown. The X-ray tube used in SOMATOM has a particularly long life, and – assuming an average of 15 examinations per day – frequently remains in operation for over six months.

Simplicity of Service

When a CT system breaks down, the problem must be located and corrected as quickly as possible. Here, the computer can function as a troubleshooting aid: operational error messages can be outputted automatically, so that the service technician can quickly determine the cause of the problem. The Siemens CT system concept permits rapid troubleshooting as a result of comprehensive test programs, the use of similar component groups and accessibility. This reduces repair time to a minimum.

4.2 Uniformity of the Technical Concept

The decision to purchase a particular CT system is far-reaching for both the buyer and the operator. This concerns above all the cost of acquisition. Equally important are the follow-up costs for maintenance and routine operation.

Overhauling a system already installed or purchasing an additional system are, for reasons of cost, only possible after a time of several years has elapsed. Some general considerations to aid in the decision to purchase a particular CT system are:

▷ system performance
▷ reliability of manufacturer
▷ speed of servicing
▷ guaranteed availability of spare parts over an extended period of time
▷ continual product improvement
▷ state-of-the art technology
▷ high standard of quality

A comparison of the technical data for different systems is in itself not enough to decide which system to purchase, because these data only reflect the situation of the moment. The experience of the manufacturer in medical technology, particularly in X-ray technology and other imaging methods, and the capability to guarantee the functioning of the CT system over several years are also important considerations (Fig. 4.3).

Numerous manufacturers of CT systems developed and marketed their equipment during the initial phase of computed tomography. Some failed, however, to live up to the routine demands of clinical practice. Design concepts of great interest were unable to gain a foothold, because these systems were not able to live up to the extremely rigorous operational demands expected of them. The high level of investment on the part of some manufacturers for a technical service organization located near the customer and for the continual routine servicing of the systems installed made it impossible for these firms to function on a cost-

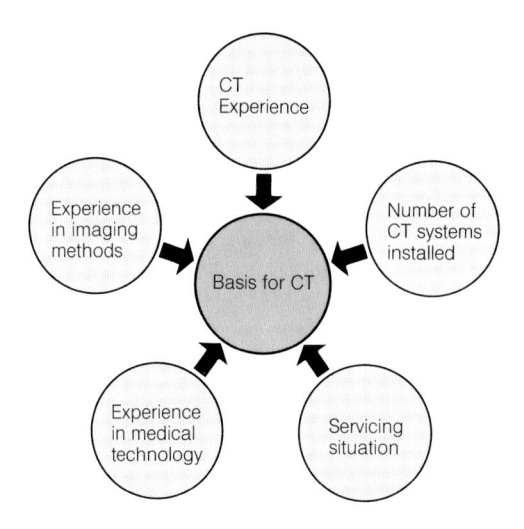

Fig. 4.3
A few important considerations for evaluating the performance of a CT manufacturer

effective basis. The result was that such manufacturers disappeared from the CT market and the user was then faced with the unpleasant situation of still having guaranteed service without being able to take advantage of future CT developments. This situation made it impossible to maintain state-of-the-art technology and to participate in the newer developments in computed tomography.

System components

As already indicated, an important step in selecting a CT system is a consideration of its system components. Siemens develops and manufactures its own system components, thus providing optimal interaction between these components. These include:

X-ray tube and generator
detector system with electronics
computer and software
mechanical components and patient table

X-ray tube and generator

Since the installation of an X-ray tube entails not only costs, but also downtime, the life of the X-ray tube is very important. The X-ray tube is, as in any other X-ray system, a part which wears with time. Since the requirements imposed on this component in computed tomography are much more demanding than in conventional X-ray equipment, only specially developed heavy duty tubes are suitable for operation in a CT system. The heat storage capacity of the anode plate and the cooling rate of the X-ray housing are the factors which determine long-term performance, peak loading and, as a result, the operating speed and reliability of the system.

This assumes particular importance, for example, in examinations of the inner ear in very thin slices, requiring a high level of tube loading. Unless the X-ray tube has a reserve loading capacity, waiting times for the tube to cool down are unavoidable. The same applies to the serial techniques discussed in Chapter 3, which excel in being able to perform fast scanning sequences.

A high-voltage generator matched to the X-ray tube must be able to provide an adequate output level for the examination procedure. Only the high-output generators known from conventional X-ray diagnostics are able to fulfil the extreme demands of computed tomography. Examples of these are to be found in cine-angiography or the most recent special units developed for use with CT systems.

Detector system with electronics

Another important system component is the detector. Its material and design determine the efficiency for detecting incident X-radiation. The dimensions and the arrangement of its individual elements decisively influence the resolution capability which can be attained. The combination of scintillation crystals with photodiodes and high-pressure inert gas detectors used in SOMATOM is of practical significance. Both detector systems produce CT images of the highest quality. Decisive for the quality, however, is not so much the type of detector as the experience and understanding of the technology required for its manufacture, along with its reliability in everyday operation.

Computer and Software

The design of a CT system computer determines, in addition to functional reliability and flexibility, the waiting time for a CT image. With SOMATOM, today's technology allows the reconstruction of even 512 x 512 image matrices during the course of the CT scan.

The typical array processors used for image construction are generally not optimized for the reconstruction of CT images. Only a high speed computer with extremely fast reconstruction times, developed especially for this purpose, is equal to the task. The host computer of a CT system is responsible for essentially different tasks. It must supervise data files, control the entire system, process operating commands from different input devices and be suitable for connection to memory arrays of the most varied types. A flexible operating system for the host computer which has been well tested under practical conditions is then decisive. Peak performance in computed tomography is only possible today with such separate systems, since both computers can then be optimally matched to the requirements of the examination.

The software used for acquiring and diagnosing CT images belongs to a wide-ranging software system, which – in addition to operating the system – also includes system monitoring and adjustment. This "tailor made" software system for each system type is being continually extended and improved; simple and comfortable operation are to a great extent the result of high performance capability.

Mechanical Components and Patient Positioning

Scanning times in the range of a few seconds make great demands on the drive mechanism. Jolt-free startup, noiseless rotation and damped braking are all important in this regard.

Absolutely essential to achieve these aims are ball bearings and a robust, long wearing drive mechanism. Along with these, there must be an angle of inclination for the scanning unit sufficient to permit stepwise oblique scanning.

The examination of traumatized or immobile patients is becoming increasingly more important. This requires matching the patient table to all possible bed heights and, in particular, moving the patient couch to very low levels. These requirements are thus similar to those for classical X-ray diagnostics. Since the patient table and suitable positioning aids are decisive in determining the possible number of examinations which can be performed with a CT system, manufacturers with experience in other fields of X-ray diagnostics and in clinical practice are better able to offer a suitable design (Fig. 4.4).

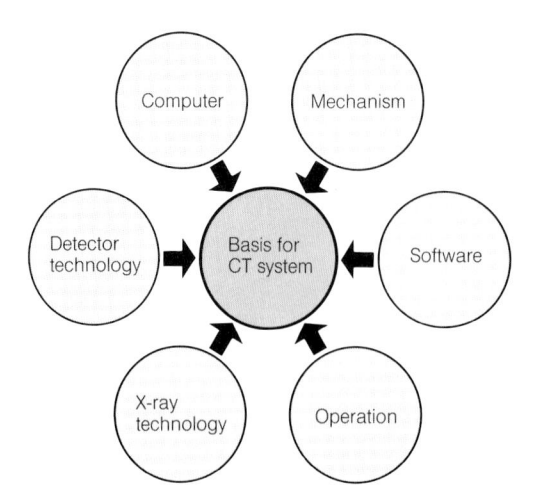

Fig. 4.4
Technological considerations having a decisive influence on performance and reliability of a CT system

Component Compatibility and the System Concept

As with any other technical system, a CT system represents a compromise between cost and available technology. While the separate consideration of the individual components is important in its own right, it does not suffice to give a comprehensive description of the standard of performance. Equally as important is the optimization of the system components relative to each other and the level of optimization achieved in the performance of the individual components. Only then is the interplay of components satisfactory and their operation reliable. As an example for this interplay, the effects of an abbreviated scanning time are considered: first, the X-ray tube and generator must offer a high level of performance over the abbreviated scanning time. However, a higher X-ray tube output necessitates more efficient heat dissipation, since for an abbreviated scanning time the individual scans of the sequence are triggered earlier. Scan values accumulate quickly, so that the electronics must be equal to the task of data acquisition. In order not to lose the advantage of shorter scanning times by having to endure waiting times, the image reconstruction must proceed faster, while at the same time images already produced must be stored faster into the applicable memories. Higher rotational speeds occur during rotary operation of the system, giving rise to greater forces of acceleration, which in turn must be taken into account in the system design. And finally, operation and documentation of the patient scans onto film must also take place at an increased speed.

This example demonstrates that the optimization of a CT system makes modifications necessary in the components which most heavily determine the system performance level, unless these components are all part of a well considered system concept. Such a system comes about only as a result of developing, testing and improving the entire system and the interplay of its components.

4.3 Add-on Capability

Owing to the high costs invested, a very important aspect of purchasing a CT system is how easily the system can be updated to meet future requirements. Experience during the initial phase of computer tomography confirms this: the pace of developments in this period made many systems outdated within the short time of a few years. A modern CT scanner must therefore allow for future expansion and improvement.

Component Principle

In most clinics, a CT unit is used today as a universal installation. This implies that the selection of a CT system must take into account the needs and wishes of all the various X-ray diagnostic groups. A meaningful way to adapt the CT system to the equipment already in place and to the requirements of the individual

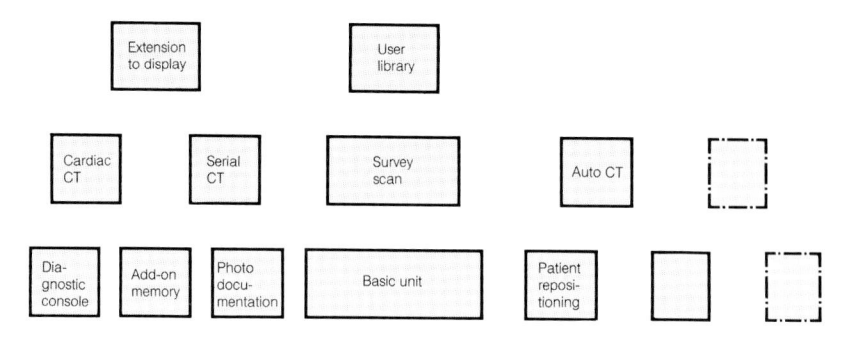

```
┌──────────────┐                    ┌──────────────┐
│  Extension   │                    │    User      │
│  to display  │                    │   library    │
└──────────────┘                    └──────────────┘

┌──────────┐  ┌──────────┐  ┌──────────────┐            ┌──────────────┐   ┌ ─ ─ ─ ┐
│ Cardiac  │  │  Serial  │  │    Survey    │            │   Auto CT    │   │       │
│   CT     │  │    CT    │  │    scan      │            │              │   │       │
└──────────┘  └──────────┘  └──────────────┘            └──────────────┘   └ ─ ─ ─ ┘

┌──────┐ ┌──────┐ ┌──────┐ ┌────────────────┐  ┌──────────┐            ┌ ─ ─ ─ ┐
│ Dia- │ │Add-on│ │Photo │ │                │  │ Patient  │            │       │
│gnostic│ │memory│ │docu- │ │   Basic unit   │  │ reposi-  │            │       │
│console│ │      │ │menta-│ │                │  │ tioning  │            │       │
└──────┘ └──────┘ │ tion │ └────────────────┘  └──────────┘            └ ─ ─ ─ ┘
                  └──────┘
```

Fig. 4.5a
Components of a CT system. Possibilities for adding on to the basic unit, illustrated for SOMATOM.

clinic is to divide the system into a basic unit and additional extensions. Even if at the time of acquiring a CT system only the normal standard operation is planned, the user should consider if all known components or components expected to be available within the foreseeable future for the system can be supplied. In keeping with today's standard, a modern CT system must be able to expand to include the extension to digital survey scans, dynamic computed tomography, reconstructing coronal, sagittal or oblique slices from transaxial slices, and for the extension to a therapy planning system. Furthermore, even now there are already extensions for cardiac CT examinations (making use of ECG for slices coordinated with cardiac phase) or software extensions to permit a semi-automatic examination sequence. All in all, the concept to be preferred is that which allows the greatest freedom for future expansion. This is greatly facilitated by the presence of the applicable interfaces and components. The CT system with a largely modular construction already takes this into account. A system conceived with a view to the future and for long-term service is therefore sufficiently flexible for adaption to the performance level and the clinical requirements expected.

Moreover, a system designed in this manner offers the assurance that, even after a longer time has elapsed, new developments can still be accommodated (Fig. 4.5).

Computer Software

Particularly important for the cost-effective operation of a modern CT system are the extensive programs for control, scanning, image reconstruction and image evaluation. Since these can be replaced, CT system users have the opportunity

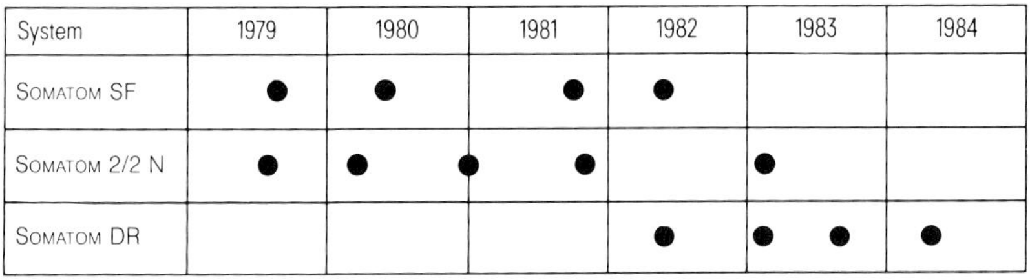

System	1979	1980	1981	1982	1983	1984
SOMATOM SF	●	●		●	●		
SOMATOM 2/2 N	●	●	●	●		●	
SOMATOM DR				●	●	●	●

Fig. 4.5 b
Example of product updating: important software improvements for three SOMATOM systems

to assimilate all future improvements and extensions. In fact, most developments in computed tomography over the past few years have become available to a wide circle of users in just this way. A typical example of this is the enhancement of resolution through the use of special algorithms, as was discussed in chapter 3. The resulting substantial extension of the range of application for a CT scanner was made available to the users in the form of updated software (Fig. 4.5a) – mostly without having to carry out any hardware alterations.

4.4 Standard of Quality

In order for a CT scanner to operate reliably over a long period, steps must be taken to guarantee a high standard of quality. The most important steps reponsible for quality and reliability are:

product concept and development
manufacture
installation at user location
servicing

During all these steps, reproducible quality must be consciously stressed from the very beginning (Fig. 4.6).

Using the example of a modern whole-body scanner, the SOMATOM, we will discuss some of these measures and the effort allotted to them.

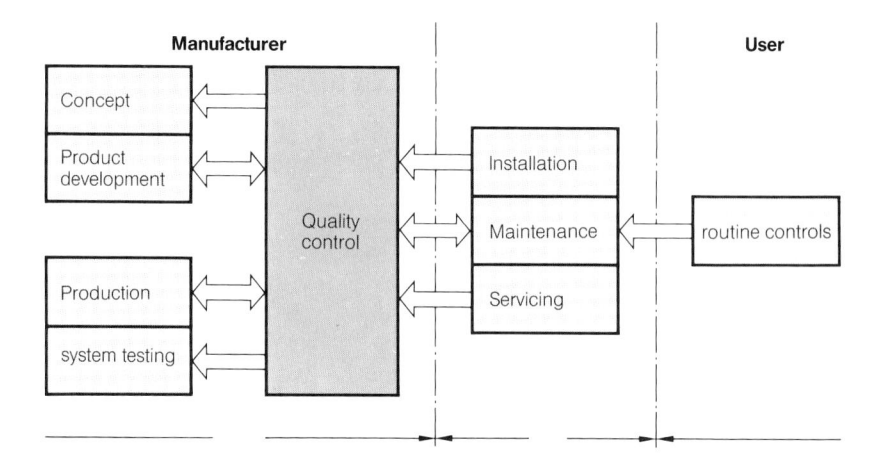

Fig. 4.6
Quality control and assurance: typical stations on the way to continuous monitoring of quality

Planned Quality

As early as during the development phase of such a system, decisions are made in regard to reliability and reproducibility which have far reaching implications for design and construction. It was possible with the X-ray components to fall back on many years of experience. This is particularly advantageous in regard to the high-output X-ray tube with the high-performance compound anodes constructed of tungsten, alloyed with rhenium, molybdenum and graphite. The proven life of these X-ray tubes, used in hundreds of SOMATOM installations for many years, speaks well for the correctness of the principle of construction. In regard to the generator, it was possible to call upon extensive knowledge and experience with high-output generators in the field of cine-angiography. The result was a new generator with "the most modern high-frequency technology", tailor made for CT operation.

The detector construction assumes a high level of technical competence. Only by means of parallel investigations into the alternative methods (crystal with photomultiplier, high-pressure ionization chambers or crystal with semiconductors) and their performance in regard to efficiency, life cycle, insensitiveness to disturbances and mechanical stability is it possible to decide upon the optimum detector system.

The computer components must satisfy the high demands of speed, flexibility and the capacity to assimilate add-on memory.

Table 4.1
Extent of scanning and troubleshooting programs for SOMATOM. Testing and adjusting the system require more effort than a patient scan.

Type of program	Number of commands
Scanning program	118,912
Troubleshooting program	81,664
Adjustment program	76,160

Specialized research in our own image reconstruction laboratory permit putting experience dating back to the 1974 version of SIRETOM into practice. This demonstrated the wisdom of assigning device control and data supervision to a well-proven host computer and image reconstruction to a high-speed computer. The same laboratory also carried out long-term performance testing of the mechanical and electronic components under unfavorable environmental conditions.

The extensive range of computer programs for adjustment and functional testing remains largely oblivious to the operator. These programs are, however, essential for the continuous quality control of the CT system. For the SOMATOM whole-body scanner, by way of example, these programs are more extensive than those for scanning and reconstruction. Along with the extension and improvement of the scanning programs, the adjustment and troubleshooting programs are also updated. This allows finer testing criteria to reach all operating installations through regular routine servicing (Table 4.1).

Production and Final System Checkout

During manufacture and installation of SOMATOM, a wide-ranging network of controls and functional checks insures a uniformly high level of quality. Incoming materials and construction elements used in the manufacture of a CT system undergo very strict checkout controls. All electronic components are subjected to individual checkout procedures prior to assembly. The larger parts, such as the generator, X-ray tube, patient table, operating console, computer etc. are only released for final assembly after undergoing exhaustive final checkout procedures.

During testing, computed tomography systems are installed just as will be done at the user's facility. Each system is then checked out in great detail and adjusted with great care during a testing procedure which lasts several weeks. Of particular importance here are the precise adjustment of the beam, collimators and detector in relation to each other, an image quality test and the testing of electrical and

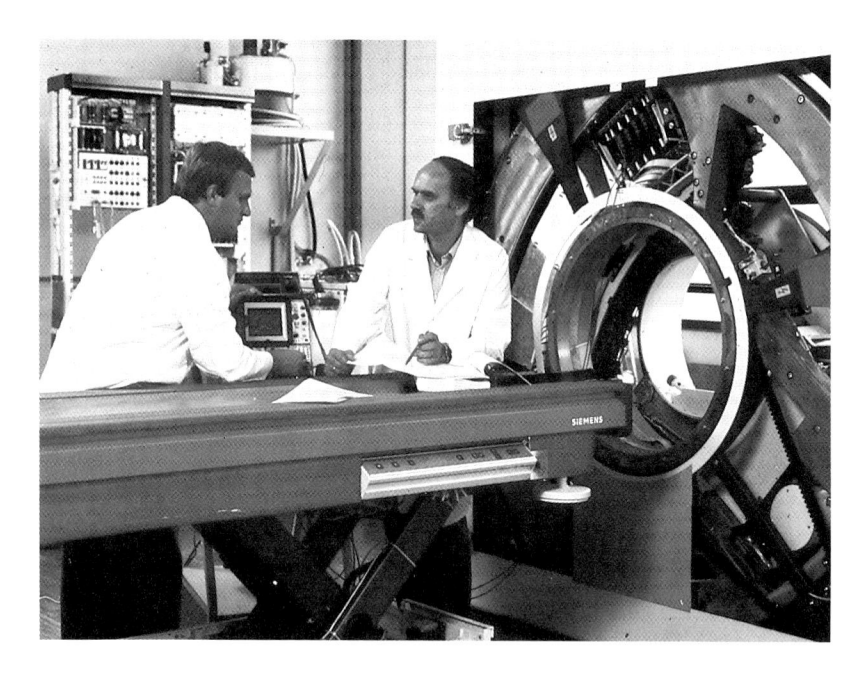

Fig. 4.7   Final system checkout for a SOMATOM

mechanical reliability. When the required quality level has been attained and the system functions error-free, all settings are entered in a test protocol and a set of test images is generated. These test documents then remain with the system (Fig. 4.7).

Installation and Functional Checkout

After delivery and installation of the SOMATOM at the clinic, the quality testing is repeated on-site. Only after all operational values in the test protocol have been reproduced and have stabilized is the system released for routine operation. The documentation on the system status after turnover and the first patient scans are evaluated at the factory and stored in computer memory. During the first week of operation, a specially trained engineer monitors system performance.

Routine operation begins only following this procedure (Protocol 4.1).

```
SOMATOM DR ADJUSTMENT STATUS AND DETECTOR PROPERTIES REPORT
============================================================

SOMATOM DR2
     -18810      VERSION NUMBER
          0      GENERATOR  ( 0 = PANDOROS / 1 = MIKROMATIC )
        256      MATRIX
       1194                        EQUIPMENT SERIAL NUMBER
  18-APR-83      TUNING DATE
       1131      GENERATOR SERIAL NUMBER
  18-APR-83      TUNING DATE
       3226      DETECTOR SERIAL NUMBER
  18-APR-83      TUNING DATE
          1      NUMBER OF X-RAY TUBES
     526871      X-RAY TUBE SERIAL NUMBER
          0      NUMBER OF SCANS
  18-APR-83      TUNING DATE


        DL0      SYSTEM UNIT
        DR0      UNIT INSTALLED
        DR1      UNIT INSTALLED
        DY0      UNIT INSTALLED
        DY1      UNIT INSTALLED

VALUES OF SLICE 1-3
===================
          2      NOMINAL VALUE OF SLICE 1
         21      VALUE OF TUBE DIAPHRAGM
         30      VALUE OF DETECTOR DIAPHRAGM
          4      NOMINAL VALUE OF SLICE 2
         32      VALUE OF TUBE DIAPHRAGM
         60      VALUE OF DETECTOR DIAPHRAGM
          8      NOMINAL VALUE OF SLICE 3
         55      VALUE OF TUBE DIAPHRAGM
        119      VALUE OF DETECTOR DIAPHRAGM

RESULTS OF AXIAL X-RAY COLLIMATION
==================================

-- RESULT OF SLICE 1 (RIGHT SIDE)
EXECUTION SUCCESSFUL
PLATEAU HOMOGEN
DHHS - CONDITIONS FULFILLED
       2.02      PLATEAU LENGTH (MM)
       0.44      Z POSITION (MM)
       6.36      PLATEAU LENGTH AT 25% WIDTH (MM)
  02-MAY-83      TUNING DATE

-- RESULT OF SLICE 1 (LEFT SIDE)
EXECUTION SUCCESSFUL
PLATEAU HOMOGEN
DHHS - CONDITIONS FULFILLED
       2.34      PLATEAU LENGTH (MM)
      -0.09      Z POSITION (MM)
       6.22      PLATEAU LENGTH AT 25% WIDTH (MM)
  02-MAY-83      TUNING DATE
```

Fig. 4.8
Excerpt from a turnover protocol. The serial numbers of important components are stored and slice settings measured and recorded.

Servicing and Spare Parts

Regular routine servicing, which checks out, adjusts or replaces up to 150 components, reduces the downtime for a CT system. For the CT system user, this means an easy-to-follow picture of the expenditure in cost and time. The individual steps in routine servicing are:

▷ safety checkout
   mechanical safety
   electrical safety
   radiation shielding

▷ operational checkout
   reliability testing (see details above)
   performance and operational safety monitoring
   adjustment, settings and lubrication
   checkout of standard data and necessary corrections
   supplementing and, as necessary, replacement of auxiliary aids

▷ Maintenance and repairs
   Repair of damage and elimination of disturbances due to wear during long-term operation (except for high-vacuum parts), as well as replacement of critical parts before these can cause system downtime

A world-wide customer service network guarantees that service is always available to the user. The elimination of disturbances and routine servicing of the system are thus possible with a minimum of downtime. In addition, experienced engineers at the factory routinely examine all technical servicing reports and communications on quality testing, and all experience direct from the field is compiled at a central location. This guarantees a uniformly high quality level and permits a quick overview of the extent and nature of qualitative defects, as well as the immediate initiation of solutions (Protocol 4.2).

In order to eliminate technical disturbances as quickly as possible, entire component groups are replaced. This procedure saves valuable operating time, and the defects can be localized in a short time with the aid of the system testing programs.

The speedy elimination of defects is possible only if all spare parts are immediately available for the entire operational life of the system. A minimum complement of the most frequently needed spare parts is therefore available to the user through customer service, while the less frequently needed parts are available on short notice from the regional spare parts warehouses.

A central spare parts department at the factory also sends out parts on the same day that a TELEX order is received. In order to reduce the downtime for SOMATOM systems to a minimum, spare parts are stored at the factory, as well as at regional spare parts warehouses.

All of these measures are designed to guarantee the high standard of quality for SOMATOM for the present and the future and keep downtime to a minimum. The typical SOMATOM system operates flawlessly more than 95% of the time, even when more than 25 patients are examined per day.

SIEMENS

Department of Medical Engineering
Technical Services

Preventive Maintenance: I ☐, II ☐, III ☐   Checklist: _____

SOMATOM DR1 / DR2 / DR3 / DRG / DRH   Page: 1–8

Manufacturing-No.: _____

I	II	III	Maintenance interval:	Months	Preventive maintenance	Months	Preventive maintenance	In order or adjusted	Part must be replaced
				1	I	7	I		
				2	I	8	I		
				3	I	9	I		
				4	I	10	I		
				5	I	11	I		
				6	II	12	III		

A. Safety checks

1. Mechanical safety

I	II	III		In order	Part
X	X	X	1.1. Check function of all emergency-off buttons (on-site)	O	O
X	X	X	1.2. Check that all radiation protection components are installed on the control assembly (Pandoros CT3 only)	O	O
		X	1.3. Check gantry safety system – rotation stop	O	O

2. Electrical safety

X	X	X	2.1. Check function shutdown during table movement	O	O
	X	X	2.2. Check safety switch:		
			– tilt	O	O
			– table feed	O	O
			– lift	O	O
X	X	X	2.3. Check measurement of protective ground conductor	O	O
		X	2.4. Check high-voltage monitoring (Pandoros CT3 only)	O	O

3. Radiation protection

X	X	X	3.1. Check radiation shutdown for emergency stop (on the unit)	O	O
X	X	X	3.2. Check radiation shutdown for computer failure	O	O

4. Multispot M

| | | X | – see separate Multispot M check list (R 57–070.102) | | |

B. Computer systems, DEC components
(This work is performed in the course of the computer maintenance)

PDP 11/44 or PDP 11/24

X	X	X	– Check fan function	O	O
X	X	X	– Check supply voltage REFERENCE: DC, ON – lamp on, not flashing	ACTUAL	

Fig. 4.9
Excerpt from a service protocol. Electrical reliability and radiation shielding are checked, in total about 150 points.

Literature

Deckner, R.: Wirtschaftlichkeit der Computertomographie Röntgenpraxis Bd. 33, September 1980, H. 9, pp. 208–215

Gempel, P. A.; Harris, G. H.; Evens, R. G.: Comparative Cost Analysis: Computed Tomography Versus Alternative Procedures. 1977 and 1980, Cambridge, Mass., Arthur D. Litte, Inc., 1977

Evens, R. G.: The Economics of Computed Tomography: Comparison with Other Health Care Costs. Radiology 136, pp. 509–510, August 1980

Axel, L.; Arger, P. H.; Zimmermann, R. A.: Applications of Computerized Tomography to Diagnostic Radiology. Proc. IEEE, Vol. 71, No. 3, March 1983, pp. 293–297

Evens, R. G.; Jost, R. G.: Computed Tomography Utilization and Charges in 1981 Radiology 145, pp. 427–429, November 1982

Eulow, R. A.: The Effect of the Computed Tomography Scanner on Utilization and Charges for Alternative Diagnostic Procedures. Radiology, Bd. 136, pp. 413–417, August 1980

Glossary

Absorption capability
Capability to convert radiation by means of the photoelectric effect into another form of energy. In the photoelectric effect, atomic electrons are set free due to interaction with radiation quanta. The energy imparted to the electrons can be converted into heat, for example.

ACTA Scanner
First (1973) commercial X-ray CT scanner suitable for examining the entire body, developed by Robert S. Ledley. The scanner functioned according to the → translation-rotation principle, without an → object thickness compensator.

Air calibration
See → calibration, air

Algorithm
Computational procedure, for CT to reconstruct the image from the measured → attenuation profiles. Originally, an iterative procedure was used in CT for image reconstruction, which has since given way to the so-called → convolution procedure.

Algorithm, edge-enhancing
Computational procedure accentuating contrast differences during reconstruction of the attenuation distribution giving better geometrical resolution than the standard → algorithm, but at the cost of increasing image noise.

Algorithm, high-resolution
Computational procedure for image reconstruction taking full advantage of scanning system resolution characteristics, i.e. → beam width, in order to produce an image having as great a → resolution capability as possible. In doing so, it may be necessary to accept a greater susceptibility to → artifacts as the price for improved → resolution.

Algorithm-induced noise
Signal contributions not deriving from the representation of information in the individual points of a CT image, caused by slight imprecisions in the computations required for image reconstruction.

Algorithm, standard
Computational procedure for image reconstruction without any additional smoothing or accentuation of the attenuation distribution. For the convolution procedure, this is achieved with the → convolution kernel of Shepp and Logan.

Aliasing
Superposition of signal from the region of higher spatial frequencies (beyond one half of the → scanning frequency) onto signal from the region of lower spatial frequencies in the scan obtained for the → discrete sampling of a function. It is the result of violating the → Sampling Theorem.

Aliasing artifact
→ Artifact due to violation of the → Sampling Theorem during scanning of attenuation data for a CT image. Such artifacts can occur, for example, in the form of fine streaks or a fine net in the image. See also → Aliasing.

Analog-to-digital converter (ADC)
Functional group of electronic components for converting an analog input signal, usually in the form of a voltage, into a digitally-coded output signal describing the input magnitude.

Anode
Positive electrode, such as in an electronic tube or an X-ray tube. For X-ray tubes, there is a distinction between → stationary anode tubes and → rotating anode tubes.

Anode, inherent filtration of
When the anode of an X-ray tube shows → roughening after having been in service over a long time or due to overloading, the X-radiation originating from the more deeply lying regions of the rough anode surface is at least partially filtered in passing through the higher-lying anode regions. This filtering leads to a change in the spectral composition of the X-radiation which the tube produces.

Anode loading capacity
Permissible limiting value of the electrical power for electron current flowing between the cathode and anode of an X-ray tube. The permissible instantaneous power is determined essentially by the melting point of the anode material. It is for the most part a function of anode temperature, current density (focal spot size when the current is given) and the interaction time of the electron beam on the anode. The permissible average power over short periods of time, such as for a single scan series, is determined largely by the heat storage capacity of the anode, while over longer periods of time, such as hours, it is limited by the dissipation of heat from the anode to its environment. See → rotating anode tube, → stationary anode tube, → anode, metal-graphite.

Anode, metal-graphite
Rotating anode for X-ray tubes, consisting of a metal plate and a thick graphite disc soldered together. The addition of the graphite disc greatly increases both the heat loading capacity and the heat radiating capability of the anode.

Anode, monitoring of loading
The state of loading for the anode of an X-ray tube can be controlled by non-contact measurement of the anode temperature. For a CT system, such monitoring can be performed by the system computer, since it can determine the given anode temperature and the loading which is still permissible from the data for previous tube operation and the known heat-up and cool-down behavior of the anode.

Anode roughening
When electrons impinge upon the anode of an X-ray tube, this can result in surface temperatures high enough to melt the anode surface. After the anode has been operating over a long time or when it is operated at a high but unsteady beam output, a roughening of the surface results which gives rise to a noticeable change in the X-ray spectrum generated and which can lead to a worsening of the X-ray tube efficiency. See → anode, inherent filtration, above.

Anti-scatter collimation
Reduction of scattered radiation contribution to X-radiation incident upon → detector input by means of a suitable → collimator. See also → Groedel technique.

Area noise
Fluctuations in the average CT number values within preselected (usually circular) test areas in the image of a homogeneous phantom, arising from quantum → noise, electronic → noise and → algorithm-induced noise. The → standard deviation of the average CT number value is most often given as a measure of area noise for a preselected test area size. The area noise for a definite test area size determines for what level of contrast an object detail of corresponding cross-section can be represented in a homogeneous environment under the same scan conditions (Object size, → attenuation capability, scan parameters).

Array
1. One- or multi-dimensional data or numerical field, such as in computer memory.
2. One- or two-dimensional arrangement of the same elements, such as the arrangement of detector elements into a detector array.

Array processor
Computer constructed and organized so that it can perform special mathematical operations on numerical fields at particularly high speed.

Artifact
Component of an image having no counterpart in the distribution of the physical parameter of the object to be imaged. In a CT image, both structure artifacts and attenuation value falsifications (→ CT number falsifications) can appear as artifacts.

Artifact, aliasing
See → aliasing artifact.

Artifact, beam hardening
Falsification of structure and/or → CT number values as a result of errors in measurement caused by changes in the X-ray beam spectrum in passing through the object being examined (→ beam hardening error). → Beam hardening artifacts can occur in the image when the → attenuation properties of the object deviate significantly from the assumptions underlying the → beam hardening correction.

Artifact behavior
Way in which an imaging artifact arises.

Artifact, motion (-induced)
Imaging error arising from motion of the object during scanning. In a CT image, such movements do not lead to blurring at the edge as in a classical X-ray image, but to wide-ranging → artifacts.

Artifact, partial volume

→ Artifact caused by pronounced material inhomogeneities (such as with bone-air transitions) within a scanning → beam. The linear → attenuation coefficient, μ, the object material property most directly imaged in CT, the object thickness, d, and the beam intensities, J (with object) and J_0 (with no object in the beam path), are related by $\mu \cdot d = \ln J_0 - \ln J$.
Each detector element averages the intensity in the corresponding beam, but not the logarithm of the intensity, as required by the relation above. Therefore, scan data discrepancies, which may show up in the form of artifacts, can arise between beams which penetrate inhomogeneous material along different paths.

Artifact, ring-shaped
CT image artifact concentric to the imaging point of the → system axis. In → fan-beam scanners with a rotating detector system, it can be caused by minute deviations in the absorption behavior of neighboring detector elements. With → translation-rotation scanners and → ring-detector scanners, it can be caused by periodic beam intensity fluctuations occurring synchronously with motion of the scanner or sampling of detector signals.

Assembler
Programming language which allows programming a computer at the level of the individual arithmetic unit commands.

Attenuation capability
See → beam attenuation capability.

Attenuation coefficient, linear
See → attenuation, law of.

Attenuation, law of
The functional relationship between the radiation intensity, J, behind an absorbing homogeneous object of thickness d and the intensity, J_0, which would be measured at the same position if the object were not in the path of the beam:

$$J = J_0 e^{-\mu d}$$

This relationship is also known as Beer's Law and is valid in the simple form given here only for monochromatic X-radiation (i.e., X-radiation having only quanta of a single energy) and for a narrow beam, in which scattered radiation can be neglected. The constant μ is designated the linear attenuation coefficient.

Attenuation profile
Spatial distribution of total attenuation in the slice under investigation, in a particular projection direction.

Attenuation properties
All properties characterizing the → beam attenuation capacity.

Automatic zeroing
See automatic → offset adjustment

Background
Program level having lower priority during program execution with a computer for which the operating system permits simultaneously running two programs of different priorities. See also → foreground.

Back projection
Computation of individual contributions of measured and convolved (see → convolution) → attenuation profiles to the individual picture elements.

Bar test
Test phantom for determination of → resolution capability, preferably a cylinder made of acrylic glass or some other plastic material, containing inserts provided with grooves of rectangular cross-section arranged parallel to each other and to the axis of the cylinder. These grooves are arranged in rows, so that in any given row all grooves have the same width and the distance between the centers of adjacent grooves is twice this width. Corresponding arrangements of small plastic sheets are sometimes used in place of the grooves.

Beam attenuation capacity
Capacity to reduce the intensity of X-radiation by absorption and scattering.

Beam filtration
Installation of additional beam filters in beam path between the X-ray tube and object to be scanned. Beam filtration has the effect of reducing low-energy components in the X-ray spectrum. Since these spectral components are largely absorbed by the scan object in any case, this results in a lower → patient dose level for the same detector signal level. Also, beam hardening by the scan object is less pronounced. This in turn makes the → beam hardening correction simpler and reduces the occurrence of → beam hardening artifacts.

Beam hardening correction
Compensation for errors in measurement arising from changes in the X-ray spectrum caused by penetrating the object scanned (→ beam hardening errors) by means of corresponding correction of scan data. The correction assumes that the change in spectrum during penetration of the scanning object differs only insignificantly from that resulting through penetration of a homogeneous standard object. See also → dual-energy method.

Beam hardening effect
Change in spectrum of a polychromatic X-ray beam, such as the Bremsstrahlung used in X-ray diagnostics, during penetration of an absorbing substance. Since the low-energy spectral components (with the exception of absorption edges) are always attenuated more strongly than the high-energy components, the energy distribution of the spectrum is displaced toward higher energy values. The penetration capability of the X-radiation then increases. In other words, the beam becomes "harder".

Beam hardening error
Error in measurement during determination of → beam attenuation capacity, resulting from change in X-ray spectrum due to penetration of the scan object. The change is the result of stronger attenuation of the low-energy spectral components, compared with the higher-energy components. Its effect is that, for the same material, increasing object thickness gives rise to a decrease in attenuation capability relative to the object thickness in the beam direction.

Beam quality
Spectral composition of an X-ray beam. The beam quality is determined by the high voltage of the X-ray tube, anode material, anode condition, filters in the beam path and possibly by the scanning object.

Beam width
Effective width of beam used for determination of an attenuation value in slice

plane perpendicular to direction of beam. The beam width is determined by the → system geometry, the → focal spot size, the → focal path and the → detector element dimensions. See also → measuring beam.

Blurring, motion-induced
See motion (-induced) → artifact.

Bore hole test
Test → phantom for determination of → limiting resolution or → low-contrast resolution capability, usually a cylinder made of acrylic glass or another plastic with holes bored parallel to the cylinder axis and oriented toward each other. The holes are arranged in rows, such that all holes in the same row have the same diameter, and the distance between centers of adjacent bore holes is twice their diameter. With the versions used to determine → low-contrast resolution capability or the → contrast-detail diagram, the contrast between bore holes and basic phantom material can be varied by filling the bore holes with different fluids.

Breathing artifact
→ Motion artifact caused by chest movement.

BSP 11
Special-purpose, programmable computer, especially suited to needs of data acquisition, scan data correction and image reconstruction for computed tomography. Using the convolution-back projection algorithm the BSP 11 allows on-line processing of the scan data according to the → pipeline principle and thus provides an instantaneous image.

Bus
Special data transmission line connecting → central processing unit, → data storage devices and → peripheral devices of an electronic computer.

Calibration
1. Determination of → channel sensitivities for the individual channels of a CT system, e.g. by means of measurement without scan object, for the purpose of correcting scan data derived from an attenuating object.
2. Correction of scan data sets in accordance with individual → channel sensitivities.

Calibration, air
Scan performed without attenuating object in beam path, usually for purpose of → calibration or determination of individual → channel sensitivities.

Cardio CT
Representation of the heart by means of CT. Due to the rapid movements of the heart, special manipulations are necessary in order to avoid → motion artifacts. For the corresponding image reconstruction, either the beam is switched on during several CT scans only during a particular cardiac phase and only long enough to acquire enough data to reconstruct an image of the heart in this phase, or all the data from several scans are stored along with ECG data and subsequently sorted according to any desired cardiac phase, which can be selected after scanning. In both cases, the scan must be coordinated with the cardiac rhythm, so that all data for a single cardiac phase taken from different individual scans cannot accidentally be located in the same regions of angulation.

Central Processing Unit (CPU)
Central control unit of a computer, controlling and coordinating interaction of arithmetic unit, → data storage devices and → peripheral devices.

Channel sensitivity, individual
Ratio of change in output signal to change in input signal in a particular scanning channel. Due to minute differences in material and manufacturing tolerances, the individual scanning channels of a CT systems show variations in → sensitivity, which can be determined by means of an → air calibration.

153

Cinefluorography, image intensifier
X-ray procedure for the representation of rapidly occurring changes by recording the output image of an image intensifier with the aid of a cine camera. The procedure is used mostly for cardioangiography.

Collimator
Diaphragm system for narrowing an X-ray beam or reducing scattered radiation. In CT scanners, adjustable collimators are used in the → system axis direction between X-ray tube and patient and, in some scanning systems, immediately before the detector, for adjusting → slice thickness. The first serve to narrow the → dose profile to the width required for the slice thickness desired, while the second improves the → sensitivity profile (in the sense of a more nearly rectangular form). In ring-detector scanners, comb-shaped collimators are sometimes placed before the detectors to reduce the effective detector width, in order to improve the → resolution capability.
An anti-scatter collimator consists of grids as opaque as possible to radiation, directed toward the X-ray tube focus, and therefore allows the radiation originating from the → focal spot to pass unimpeded between the grids, while the scattered radiation arising in the object scanned is largely absorbed in the grids.

Compound anode
See → anode, metal-graphite

Computed radiography (CR)
X-ray projection technique making use of one- or two-dimensional → arrays of a large number of individual detectors. The individual detector output signals are digitized and the resulting image immediately stored in digital memory in the form of a → matrix.

Contrast-detail diagram
Representation of the minimum object contrast necessary to distinguish between the bores in the image from a → bore hole test for given scanning conditions, as a function of bore hole diameter. Contrast-detail diagrams must contain detailed information on the material and dimensions of the test phantom used, the slice thickness selected and the dose applied, since these values largely determine the → image noise level and are thus decisive factors in the contrast-detail diagram. See also → density value resolution capability and → low-contrast resolution capability.

Contrast, minimum
Minimum object contrast value necessary for recognition of a given image detail.

Convolution
Synthesis of a new mathematical function, g, from two given functions, f and h, according to the relation

$$g(x) = \int_{-\infty}^{+\infty} f(\tau) \cdot h(x - \tau) \, d\tau.$$

The function $h(x)$ is designated the convolution kernel. Replacing the integral by a sum permits clearly describing the convolution comprehensibly for functions of one dimension:
To calculate the function g at the point x_1, the following computational steps are necessary:
1. Mirroring the function $h(x)$ about the ordinate, giving the function $h(-x)$
2. Shifting the function $h(-x)$ through the distance x_1 along the abscissa
3. Multiplying the two functions, element by element
4. Summing the results of the multiplications

Convolution kernel
See → convolution.

Convolution algorithm
Image reconstruction algorithm, with which the measured → attenuation profiles are subjected to a convolution prior to → back projection. Through convolution, which basically corresponds to a highpass filter (i.e. enhancement of the signal for high spatial frequencies), wide-ranging blurring of individual object de-

tails are avoided, which would otherwise appear if the back projection of the measured attenuation profiles were performed immediately. The use of the convolution algorithm is essential for an → instantaneous image, i.e. image display immediately following the scan.

CT Dose Index (CTDI)
Quotient of the integral over the dose profile (e.g. in the → system axis) and the slice thickness. Strictly speaking, the integral must be determined over the limits $-\infty$ to $+\infty$. In practice, however (US specifications) the integration limits are set to 7.5 times the → slice thickness, to both sides of the central slice plane.

CT value falsification
Occurrence of CT values in a computed tomogram, which do not correspond to the attenuation coefficients present at the corresponding location in the object scanned. Such falsifications can, for example, result from an inadequate → beam hardening correction or from the application of an → edge-enhancing algorithm.

CT scanner with stationary detector
See → ring-detector scanner.

Data Acquisition System (DAS)
Electronic system for transferring detector signals to the CT system computer. Typical signal processing steps in the data acquisition system are amplification, integration, → multiplexing and → analog-to-digital conversion (digitization).

Data store
Device for holding data in digital format. Data storage devices commonly used include electronic switches (semiconductor memories), magnetic (magnetic tape, magnetic disc and floppy disc) and electro-optical (LASER disc) recording devices. For reasons of cost, semiconductor memory is used only for working → storage. Magnetic discs, magnetic tapes and LASER discs are used as → mass storage media, the last two particularly for archiving purposes. Magnetic discs and floppy discs are especially suited for the operating system and program memory. The floppy disc is of considerable importance as an archiving medium.

Decay characteristics
Behavior of output signal from a → detector or amplifier after input signal is no longer present.

DECNET
→ Software from Digital Equipment Corporation (Maynard, Massachusetts, USA) for connecting several computers through different transmission line facilities, such as telephone lines or an → ETHERNET system.

Density value determination, quantitative
Reading of → CT number values from a computed tomogram. The reading process can take place from a (partial) printout of the → image matrix or with the aid of a positioning device from an image stored in the → image display memory of the CT scanner. In the second case, as a rule it is also possible to output the average CT number values within an image region defined with the aid of the positioning device (→ ROI) in addition to a point-by-point readout.

Density value resolution capability
Capability to reproduce minute differences in density values or other differences in radiation → attenuation properties in the scan object. The density value resolution capability is determined primarily by the noise characteristics of the CT system. Since → noise depends strongly upon the dose measured by the CT system and the dose measured depends in turn upon the dose generated, the → slice thickness selected, the material properties of the scanning object and the dimensions of the scanning object, information concerning the density value resolution capability is meaningful only when given in conjunction with the information describing these parameters. See also → low-contrast resolution capability and → contrast-detail diagram.

Detector
Apparatus for measuring radiation intensities. In CT scanning systems, solid state → detectors and → inert gas detectors are used.

Detector, absorption capability of
Capability of a detector to convert (X)-radiation into light or other forms of energy (such as heat or ionization of gas molecules), thereby attenuating the radiation. See also solid state → detector, → inert gas detector and → absorption capability.

Detector chamber length
Dimension of → detector separating walls in an → inert gas detector, in direction of incident X-radiation.

Detector, effective width
Detector element width, reduced according to the imaging geometry. It is referred to the point at which the → system axis penetrates the → slice plane. See also → detector element dimensions.

Detector element dimensions
For a CT system, the cross-sectional area of a detector element perpendicular to the direction of incident radiation is a narrow rectangle, such that the narrow side is parallel to the slice plane. The narrow side determines the effective width of the → detector and thus influences the → beam width, while the long side determines the maximum → slice thickness possible.

Detector, inert gas
→ Detector for CT systems which uses an ionization chamber filled with inert gas under high pressure to measure intensity of X-radiation. As a rule, inert gas detectors for CT systems are comprised of a pressure chamber filled with xenon, in the inner part of which isolated plates directed toward the → focus are mounted and which serve as ionization chamber walls. They are connected with insulated housing bushings to the signal transmission system external to the pressure chamber.

Detector, high resolution
Detector with particularly short length along scan direction in order to achieve as narrow a → beam width as possible. The short length is achieved through the use of correspondingly narrow detector elements or through collimation. See also → collimator.

Detector, quarter shift
Arrangement of detector system for → fan-beam scanner with rotating detector such that a line from the → focus perpendicular to the → system axis is displaced by exactly one quarter of the distance between detector element centers from the plane separating the two central elements of the detector configuration. Corresponding → beams from projections in opposite directions are then displaced from each other by exactly one half the detector spacing and therefore overlap. This overlapping serves to reduce → aliasing artifacts.

Detector septum
Metal separator parallel to direction of incident X-radiation and to → system axis, between two adjacent cells of an → inert gas detector.

Detector, solid state
→ Detector made of solid material. Both pure → semiconductor detectors and combinations of → scintillation crystals and light-sensitive semiconductor diodes are employed as solid state detectors.

Detector, standard
Detector without special design features for achieving an extremely small → beam width and thus a very high spatial → resolution capability

Diagnostic main console (DMC)
Main control console of the SOMATOM CT system. The DMC makes scanning, archiving and evaluation of computed tomograms possible, including → image reconstruction from raw data already stored. See also → diagnostic satellite console.

Diagnostic satellite console (DSC)
Diagnostic control console of the SOMATOM CT system. The DSC makes archiving and evaluation of computed tomograms possible, including → image reconstruction from raw data already stored. See also → diagnostic main console.

Dialog monitor
See → text monitor.

Diameter, limiting
Smallest bore diameter in a → bore hole test for which the individual bore holes can still be distinguished under given scanning conditions. See also → resolution limit and → limiting geometrical resolution.

Digital radiography
X-ray projection technique with digital image scanning and processing. The radiographs are initially produced by analog methods. In general, image intensifier TV-flouroscopic images are digitized, stored in digital format and processed further. However, conventional film radiographs can also be digitized.

Digital survey scan (with CT systems)
Projection radiogram (similar to a conventional radiograph) produced by piecing rows of projections together. Between acquisition of successive scan projections the scanning system, consisting of → X-ray tube and → detector, remains in the same position. The scanning object is advanced along the → system axis. Such survey scans are possible only with → fan-beam, → hybrid and ring-detector scanners. Whereas a conventional radiograph yields a pure central projection, the digital survey scan with a CT system gives a central projection in the fan direction and a parallel projection in the direction of the system axis.

Digital-to-analog converter (DAC)
Electronic device for converting a digital signal into an analog electrical signal, usually in the form of a voltage, which in its magnitude is proportional to the input signal.

Doping
Implantation of foreign atoms into the crystal lattice of a high purity crystalline substance. With fluorescent materials, suitable doping can considerably enhance the luminous efficiency. At the same time, doping frequently leads to a worsening of → decay characteristics.

Dose, applicable
Radiation dose permissible or acceptable according to careful assessment of the risk to a patient's health for a given examination.

Dose distribution
Spatial distribution of dose values in the slice plane. The drop in dose value from the surface of the body to the inside of the body in CT differs considerably from that of classical radiographs. Since in CT the X-ray source rotates about the object scanned, as opposed to classical radiography, the direction of incident radiation changes continuously during the course of the scan. As a result, in CT the ratio of → skin dose to dose at the axis of the body is considerably lower.

Dose, patient
See → patient dose level

Dose profile
Spatial variation of dose values in the direction of the → system axis at a preselected location in the slice (usually on the system axis). Due to scattered radiation, the dose profile is always broader than the → sensitivity profile, even when there is no slice collimation between scan object and → detector.

Dose utilization
Fraction of total incident radiation energy at the detector entrance level absorbed by the → detector. The dose utilization is determined by the geometrical → dose utilization and the → absorption capability of the detector elements.

Dose utilization, geometrical
Fraction of total incident radiation energy at the detector entrance level impinging

upon the active volume of the → detector. The geometrical dose utilization is determined primarily by the → collimators at the detector and through inactive zones between adjacent detector elements resulting from the detector construction.

Double-window technique
Simultaneous display of two partial CT number regions selected from a computed tomogram, with full range of brightness for the → image monitor. This permits simultaneous viewing of image regions having widely varying average CT values (a similar situation applies to color displays). The double-window technique has proven particularly useful for displaying computed tomograms of the thorax. See also → window display.

Dual-energy method
CT procedure based on scanning of the same slice with two different X-ray beam spectra. The scan data pairs obtained for every single beam position yield information on the composition (effective atomic number) of the material in the beam path. This information permits carrying out such tasks as determining mineral content in bone, reconstructing images as would be possible with monochromatic X-radiation of freely selectable energy, and complete correction of → beam hardening effects.

ECG-gated image reconstruction
See → CARDIO CT.

Edge response function
Image of a discontinuity in density values along a plane perpendicular to the slice plane, between two homogeneous object regions. The determination of the edge response function is possible, for example, by means of the computed tomogram of a homogeneous plastic object in a water phantom. The test body must have at least one plane boundary surface running perpendicular to the slice plane during scanning.

EMI scanner
First commercial CT scanner, manufactured by EMI (Electrical and Musical Industries, Hayes, Middlesex, England). This head scanner, introduced in 1972 and having an image matrix of 80×80 elements, functioned according to the → translation-rotation principle and had a water-filled → object thickness compensator.

Energy response characteristic
Dependence of a property, e.g. → sensitivity of a → detector, on X-ray quantum energy.

Entrance window
Input area of a → detector or arrangement of detectors presented to incident X-radiation.

ETHERNET
Standardized communications system with a high data transfer rate, for connecting several computers by means of a high frequency line.

Exposure time
Time during which the scanning object is exposed to X-radiation. The exposure time is in general less than the → scanning time, especially for CT scanners having pulsed beams.

Fan-beam scanner
CT scanner which scans the entire cross section of the object under study by means of a fan-shaped beam, so that only a purely rotational motion of the X-ray source is necessary. There are fan-beam scanners having a stationary detector ring (the so-called → ring-detector scanners) as well as scanners for which an arc-shaped detector configuration rotates along with the X-ray tube about the object. The latter type of CT system is often described in short as "fan-beam scanner", in contrast to "ring-detector scanner".

Filtration, inherent
All filtration of the X-ray beam emerging from an X-ray tube assembly which arises from components of this assembly (anode,

tube glass, cooling oil, beam exit window, permanently installed filters, etc.). Inherent filtration is generally described in values of equivalent aluminum thicknesses.

Fluorescent substance
Substance which emits light as a result of interaction with radiation.

Focal spot dimensions of a CT X-ray tube
The electronic → focal spot is in general a rectangle extending much further in the radial direction (relative to the anode) than in the azimuthal direction. However, the X-ray tube is built into the CT system so that the effective optical → focal spot is seen as a square from the center of the → detector. A very small focal spot is not necessarily desirable in CT. In order to reduce → aliasing artifacts, an increased contribution from the focal spot to the → beam width can be useful.

Focal path
Spatial path which → focus executes during scanning procedure for determination of an attenuation value. See also → beam width.

Focal spot of an X-ray tube
Anode region in which X-radiation is produced through bombardment from the electron beam which the cathode generates. See also electronic → focal spot, optical → focal spot and effective optical → focal spot.

Focal spot, effective optical, of an X-ray tube
Projection of the electronic focal spot parallel to the beam passing from the → focus through the object (or detector element) of interest onto the image target area (or detector → entrance window).

Focal spot, electronic, of an X-ray tube
Area of intersection between anode surface and electron → beam produced by the cathode.

Focal spot, optical, of an X-ray tube
Projection of the electronic focal spot parallel to the beam passing from the → focus through the center of the beam exit window ("central beam") onto a plane perpendicular to this beam.

Focus of an X-ray tube
Point of concentration of the electronic → focal spot.

Foreground
Program level with greater priority during program execution for a computer in which the operating system permits running two programs of different priorities simultaneously. See also → background.

Foreground-background operation
Simultaneous execution of two programs with different priorities in a computer. See also → background and → foreground.

FORTRAN IV
Widely used higher programming language, conceived especially for the solution of mathematical, physical and technical programming problems.

Frequency, limiting
Spatial frequency at which the → modulation transfer function exhibits a definite minimum value, which the recognition of a sine wave modulation corresponding to this frequency just barely allows. The minimum value is generally not standardized and must therefore be given along with the limiting frequency in order to make a comparison between systems possible. See also → resolution limit, limiting → diameter.

Full width (at) half maximum (FWHM)
Width of a distribution at half the maximum value. See also → slice thickness and → sensitivity profile.

Gas detector
See → inert gas detector.

Generator, medium-frequency
X-ray generator in which high voltage is produced for the X-ray tube by rectifying line voltage, converting the resulting DC voltage into an AC voltage with a frequency of a few kHz, stepping up this

voltage through a transformer and then rectifying the resulting high voltage again. By comparison with the classical X-ray generator, in which the power line voltage of usually 50 or 60 Hz is immediately fed through a transformer and then rectified, this principle has the advantage of making a very much smaller transformer possible, as well as considerably improved high-voltage regulation.

Groedel technique
Radiographic technique characterized by reduction of → scattered radiation through a relatively large distance between object and image target plane.

Hardware
Collective term for all electrical and electronic switching circuitry.

High resolution detector
See → detector, high resolution.

High speed computer
Special-purpose computer, tailored to performance of particular tasks. Due to its structure, it is able to perform these tasks in a very much shorter time than a comparable, freely programmable standard computer would be able to. See also → BSP 11.

Homogeneity
The image quality property describing to what extent a test phantom of homogeneous material (such as water) is imaged with a correspondingly constant average CT number at different locations in the image.

Host computer
Computer employed for controlling and monitoring device functions, coordinating scan data acquisition and image reconstruction and controlling data transfer between the image computer and peripheral → data storage devices.

Hounsfield unit
Basic unit for the CT number scale, according to which the CT number, H, of a material is defined as 1000 times the relative deviation of the effective linear attenuation coefficient, μ, for the material from the effective linear attenuation coefficient for water, μ_w:

$$H = \frac{\mu - \mu_w}{\mu_w} \cdot 1000$$

Hybrid scanner
CT system permitting selection between two different principles for scanning the distribution of attenuation coefficients in the object slice, in particular the combination of a → translation-rotation scanner and a → fan-beam scanner with rotating → detector.

Image contrast, normalized
Quotient of the image contrast from a periodic structure – for example, a definite group of a bar test – and the image contrast resulting from the identical object contrast obtained for the same imaging system when → spatial frequency has the value zero (i.e. for structures having very large areas).

Image display memory
Electronic data storage or storage area in the CT system computer, in which the image is stored for callup as a display and from which the image can be read out at TV timing pulse rate for conversion into the analog signal required by the → image monitor.

Image, ECG-gated
See → CARDIO CT.

Image evaluation, quantitative
Any evaluation of (computertomographic) images yielding the magnitudes of particular variables, such as measurements of lengths, angles and especially density values.

Imaging geometry
Arrangement of → focal spot and → detector relative to each other and to axis of rotation for the scanning system (→ system axis) of a CT scanner. Also referred to as system geometry.

Image matrix
Two-dimensional arrangement of discrete image points (→ pixels).

Image matrix element
Individual point in an image matrix. Synonym for → pixel or image element.

Image monitor
TV viewing device for displaying a CT image. See also → text monitor.

Image noise
Image components caused by → noise.

Image reconstruction
Computational generation of an image from projection data.

Image reconstruction algorithm
See → algorithm.

Image reconstruction memory
Electronic → data storage or storage area in the CT system computer, in which the image information is stored during → image reconstruction.

Image reconstruction, secondary
Computational generation of a → secondary slice.

Image sharpness
See → resolution capability, geometrical.

Image storage, compressed
Recording of computed tomogram onto a data storage medium so as to take best advantage of the medium's information capacity. An example of this is to not store the complete CT values for the individual → image matrix elements, but instead only the differences between CT number values of adjacent elements.

Image storage, uncompressed
Recording of computed tomogram onto a → data storage medium with a defined correspondence between each data word and the corresponding → image matrix element.

Imaging, noise-free
Imaging determined only by the → modulation transfer function of the imaging system and not by signal noise or → algorithm-induced noise.

Inactive layer
Layer of a → detector in which radiation is absorbed but does not produce an output signal.

Inert gas detector
See → detector, inert gas

Instantaneous image
CT image which is available either immediately or after only insignificant delay, following termination of the CT scanning procedure.

Interface
Component making possible signal exchange between two electrical or electronic devices or component groups.

Leakage current
Very small electrical current flowing through an insulating layer.

Light intensity
Luminous current per solid angle and unit area emanating from an illuminated surface.

Line spread function (LSF)
Image of a plane running orthogonal to the slice plane. The determination of the line spread function could (by analogy to determination of the → point spread function) take place by scanning a thin metal plate spanned parallel to the → system axis, for example. But this would give rise to → artifacts, causing experimental difficulties, so that it is more expedient to obtain the line spread function by differentiation of the → edge response function.

Dose line integral
Integral over the energy dose along a line parallel to the → system axis. The quotient of the longitudinal dose product and the → slice thickness gives the dose value at the point of intersection of this line with the → slice plane for the scanning of an infinite number of adjacent slices, with the scanning parameters selected (see → CT dose index (CTDI).

Long-term power rating
See → X-ray tube power rating.

Low-contrast resolution capability
Geometrical resolution capability for minute contrast differences in the scanning object. The separation of small object structures in the image at low object contrast values depends not only on the → modulation transfer function for the CT system, but also on the → image noise, which is determined in turn by the quantum → noise and sources of noise within the system. See also → density value resolution capability and → contrast-detail diagram.

Mass storage medium
→ Data storage for large amounts of data, such as for archiving purposes. Magnetic tape, floppy disc, magnetic disc and LASER disc are all used as mass storage devices, however magnetic discs find only limited use for archiving due to their high cost.

Matching error
Geometric mismatching of two images or projections which, as a result of the scanning situation, should be identical.

Matrix
Two-dimensional set of numbers. In the context of CT, abbreviated form of → image matrix.

Measuring beam
Resultant of all primary (i.e., emanating from the X-ray tube → focal spot) X-ray beams contributing to the signal used to determine an attenuation value.

Memory
See → data storage.

Memory, working
See → data storage, working.

Microphony
Generation of undesirable signals by mechanical vibrations of electrical lines and components.

Minicomputer
Electronic computer of medium size, capacity and capability. The points of transition to a large computer or a home computer are rather diffuse and depend upon the configuration level of the individual system.

Modulation
Periodic modification of a signal, in either a temporal or spatial sense. In the context of describing → resolution capability, local variations of the attenuation pattern in the form of a sine wave (→ modulation transfer function) or a rectangle (rectangular → MTF, → bar test) are of particular importance.

Modulation transfer function (MTF, sine wave MTF)
Fourier transformation of the → point spread function. The MTF gives the relative image contrast (relative to the image contrast at zero → spatial frequency) as a function of the spatial frequency, at which a sine wave → modulation is reproduced (for constant object contrast). The MTF can be determined from the image of a wire (→ point spread function), an edge (→ edge response function, → line spread function) or a → bar test pattern (rectangular → MTF).

Monitor
TV viewing device. According to application, a distinction is made between → image monitor, → dialog monitor and → text monitor.

MTF, rectangular
The rectangular MTF is the representation of relative image contrast (relative to image contrast at zero → spatial frequency) as a function of the spatial frequency at which a rectangular-shaped modulation is reproduced (for constant object contrast). It can be determined immediately by evaluation of a → bar test scan and can be converted into the corresponding → sine wave MTF. The rectangular MTF always yields more favorable values than the sine wave MTF, because

the halfwave area under a rectangular curve is always greater than that under a sine curve of the same frequency. Consequently, only MTFs of the same kind can be compared.

Multiformat camera
Photographic camera for recording TV images onto cut film, with possibility of selecting different film format subdivision in order to record several scans onto a single film. An image monitor especially suited to photographic recording is integrated into the camera.

Multiplexing circuitry
Electronic switching circuitry permitting electrical signals of the same type from different sources to be transmitted one after another on the same transmission line. Such circuitry is used in a CT scanning system in the data acquisition system, for example, in order to transmit the output signals from different → detector elements to a common ADC.

MULTISPOT M
→ Multiformat camera with film supply magazine and receiving magazine, used with the Siemens SOMATOM. Through complete integration of this camera into the CT system software, fully automatic photographic recording of CT images is possible for one or more examinations.

Noise
Signal contributions resulting from random processes and containing no information about the variable which the signal represents.

Noise, algorithm-induced
See → algorithm-induced noise.

Noise correlation
Mutually influenced behavior of → noise in two different signals. In CT, there is a correlation e.g. for pixel → noise, i.e. the noise in one pixel is not independent of that in other pixels. The reason for this is that in CT every attenuation value measured – even if weighted differently – contributes to each pixel.

Noise, electronic
→ Noise (contribution) to electrical signals arising from electronic components.

Noise-free imaging
See → imaging, noise-free

Noise, image
See → image noise.

Noise, pixel
Fluctuation of CT values in the individual image → pixels of a homogeneous phantom or a homogeneous region of a phantom, caused by quantum → noise, electronic → noise and → algorithm-induced noise. The usual measure of pixel noise is the → standard deviation of the pixel CT values within a preselected partial region (→ region of interest (ROI) of the image. For quantitative image assessment, pixel noise by itself is of hardly any importance, since it is bound up with geometrical → resolution capability. Under otherwise identical conditions, pixel noise increases with increasing resolution.

Noise, quantum
→ Noise resulting from random processes during generation of the X-ray beam. See also → X-ray quantum.

Noise structure
Visible irregular image patterns caused by → noise.

Normalized image contrast
See → image contrast, normalized.

Nuclear medicine
Diagnosis and therapy by means of radioactive substances. For nuclear imaging procedures in medicine, radioactive substances having a relatively short half-life and often a specific affinity for single tissues are used. The substance then emits characteristic radiation which impinges upon an arrangement of detectors external to the scan object, yielding a pattern of radioactive concentration as a function of position.

Nutation
Tumbling motion of a spinning top, according to which the figure axis describes a conical shell.

Nyquist theorem
See → Sampling Theorem.

Object thickness compensator
Positioning device made of material resembling as closely as possible that of the object and shaped so that the beam paths through attenuating material are the same for all scanning beams within the slice being examined. Such devices were used with the first CT systems to reduce the dynamic range required by the detector system, as well as to largely eliminate → beam hardening errors.

Offset adjustment
Adjustment of an amplifier system to give zero output signal for zero input signal.

Offset adjustment, automatic
→ Offset adjustment of input amplifier for the detector signal performed automatically between single data readings by the CT data acquisition system.

Oil cooling
Cooling system, such as for X-ray tubes, using oil as a heat transfer medium. The oil is circulated by a pump through the object to be cooled and a heat exchanger. The heated oil is again cooled in the heat exchanger by either air or water.

Operating system
Set of all computer programs necessary for general operation of the computer and its peripheral devices.

Operating system disc
Magnetic storage disc on which the → operating system (e.g. for the CT system computer) is stored.

Partial volume artifact
See → artifact, partial volume.

Patient dose
Energy absorbed by the human body from ionizing radiation, such as X-radiation. Because of the danger of somatic or genetic damage as a result of the dose level, it is always necessary in diagnostic applications to seek a compromise between damaging effects and clinically useful information.

Peak power rating
See → X-ray tube, pulse power rating.

Peripheral device
General term for all auxiliary devices which can be connected to an electronic computer, such as user terminals, printer and magnetic disc drives.

Phantom
Scan object made of inanimate material, generally for simulating the attenuation and scatter characteristics of a biological object.

Phantom, homogeneous
Phantom with the identical composition throughout its volume.

Phantom, water
In the context of CT, usually a water-filled plastic cylinder. The vessel material should differ as little as possible from water in its attenuation characteristics. Acrylic glass is therefore used most often.

Picture (matrix) element
Individual elemental point in an image matrix.

Pile-up factor
Ratio of the maximum dose value on the scan object surface, or in the → system axis when scanning a series of adjacent object slices, and the corresponding maximum dose value for scanning a single object slice with the same parameter settings. The pile-up factor is always greater than one, since the → dose profile is always broader than the → sensitivity profile.

Pipeline principle
Execution of a sequence of data processing steps on data inputted periodically and requiring a series of arithmetic steps one after another, such that each processing

step is assigned a dedicated processor. For optimal utilization of the computational capacity, the entire data processing task is divided up into its individual steps and the single processors laid out in such a way that each of the steps can be executed in nearly the same time. This reduces the intervals between the individual processing steps to a minimum.

Pixel
See → picture (matrix) element.

Pixel noise
See → noise, pixel

Point spread function
Image of a line running perpendicular to the → slice plane. The point spread function can be determined, for example, by scanning a thin wire spanned parallel to the → system axis. The diameter of the wire should be chosen to be small relative to the expected → FWHM of the point spread function.

Program library
Compilation of data processing (sub)programs required for the solution of related problems or of a complex problem. To simplify the linking procedure for executable programs utilizing these routines, the entire set of library routines can be addressed by a single name.

Pulsed operation
Repeated switching on and off of the X-ray tube in very short regular or irregular time intervals.

Pulse energy
Energy released during the duration of an X-ray pulse. Along with the X-ray tube voltage, filtration and scanning geometry selected, the pulse energy determines the number of X-ray quanta available for each scan value measured. In order to keep the signal contribution due to electronic → noise from the → data acquisition system as low as possible for strongly attenuating objects (such as a shoulder girdle), a high pulse energy is selected in such scanning situations. For a given dose level, a better image then results with fewer projections and higher pulse energy than with more projections and lower pulse energy.

Pulse output of X-ray tube
See → X-ray tube pulse output.

Quantum
See → X-ray quantum.

Quantum noise
See → noise, quantum.

Quarter detector offset
See → detector, quarter shift.

Quarter detector shift
See → detector, quarter shift.

Reconstruction algorithm
See → algorithm.

Reconstruction center
Point in the → slice plane reproduced at the center of the image.

Reconstruction, ECG-gated
See → CARDIO CT.

Reconstruction, segmental
See → segmental reconstruction.

Region of interest (ROI)
Region of image matrix which can be selected freely in regard to position, size and form (can usually be ovelaid onto CT image) and within which special evaluation procedures, such as the computation of average CT values, can be carried out. The form selected is normally square, rectangular, circular or elliptical. For inputting an arbitrary form, generally only those forms are allowed which in a mathematical sense represent simply connected regions.

Resistor pad
Rectangular plate made from a material of relatively low conductivity, having electrical taps about its edge connected to an amplification system wired so that, when a grounded resistor pen comes into contact with the plate, output voltages proportional to the coordinates of the point touched are generated.

Resistor pen
Electronic pen for marking position in image contained in → image display memory of a CT system through a → resistor pad.

Resolution
See geometrical → resolution capability, → density value resolution capability, → low contrast resolution capability.

Resolution capability, density value
See → density value resolution capability.

Resolution capability, geometrical
Measure for the possibility of representing fine structures at (arbitrarily) high contrast level. The geometrical resolution capability is described quantitatively by the limiting geometrical → resolution, limiting- → frequency, → point spread function, → edge response function, → line response function and → modulation transfer function.

Resolution limit
Smallest value of elemental width (such as bore hole diameter or line width) for a periodic arrangement of identical individual elements, with an average center-to-center distance equal to twice the elemental width, such that the individual elements can just barely be distinguished. Alternatively, the spatial frequency corresponding to such a structure.

Resolution, limiting geometrical
→ Resolution limit for (arbitrarily) high object contrast level.

Resolution capability, low contrast
See → low contrast resolution capability.

Ring-detector scanner
→ Fan-beam scanner with a ring-shaped configuration of the individual detector elements. Most such scanners have a detector ring which remains stationary during scanning, while the X-ray tube rotates within the detector ring about the scan object. However, there are also ring-detector scanners in which the X-ray tube rotates outside of the detector ring and the detector ring executes a → nutation during scanning, so that the detector elements closest to the X-ray tube are always removed from the beam path.

Rotating anode (X-ray) tube
X-ray tube having a motor driven, disc-shaped anode which rotates rapidly about its axis. The → focal spot is located off-axis, so that it constantly changes its position on the disc during rotation. Since the anode material is therefore subjected to electron bombardment only over a short time, for given → focal spot dimensions, a rotating anode X-ray tube attains considerably higher short term power ratings than a → stationary anode X-ray tube. Cooling of the rotating anode takes place largely by means of anodic heat dissipation, so that rotating anode X-ray tubes generally show lower long-term power ratings than fluid-cooled stationary anode X-ray tubes.

Rotating operation
Operation of a → hybrid scanner as a → fan-beam scanner with rotating → detector.

Sampling, discrete
Measurement of a continuous function at individual, equidistantly separated points. See also → sampling frequency and → Sampling Theorem.

Sampling frequency
Reciprocal of the distance between the equidistant points at which the value of the function to be sampled is determined.

Sampling theorem
Mathematical principle which asserts that a continuous, band limited (i.e., not containing any spatial frequencies beyond a certain limiting frequency value) function is completely determined by its values at discrete, equidistantly located points separated by no more than one half the reciprocal of the highest spatial frequency occurring in the function. See also discrete → sampling, → sampling frequency, → aliasing.

Saturation effect
Decrease in the → sensitivity of a → detector or amplifier for a high input signal. This effect leads to a signal falsification at the output of the → detector or amplifier.

Scan data correction
Correction to the attenuation values obtained with the CT system scanning unit, in regard to → beam hardening, individual → channel sensitivity, → energy response of the individual channels and non-uniform arrangement of the individual detector elements, for example. The corrections mentioned must be performed prior to the actual → image reconstruction (such as a → convolution followed by → backprojection).

Scan field
Object space seen by input side of CT detecting system.

Scan field, central
Central part of object space seen by input side of CT detecting system. Often, special algorithms with increased memory requirements are limited in their application to the central scan field.

Scanner test
Checkout of a CT scanner in regard to definite properties or characteristic values.

Scanning frequency
Number of scans per unit time; reciprocal of scan repetition time.

Scanning properties
Characteristics of a CT scanner which determine the method of sampling the distribution of attenuation coefficients in the object slice by means of the scanning unit. These comprise → beam width, average distance between the individual → beams, → detector quarter shift and angular distance between individual projections.

Scanning time
Duration from beginning to end of scanning data acquisition for a CT scan. For most CT systems, the scanning time is greater then the → exposure time, so that it is necessary to distinguish between the two terms.

Scattered radiation
X-radiation which during interaction with matter changes in either its direction of propagation only (Rayleigh scattering, coherent scattering) or both its direction of propagation and its quantum energy (Compton scattering).

Scintillation crystal
Single crystal of a → fluorescent substance.

Secondary slice
Tomogram calculated from a series of contiguous or overlapping computed tomograms, usually with a different orientation of the slice than in the original series.

Segmental reconstruction
→ Image reconstruction for a → fan-beam scanner, using a set of projections not covering the entire angular projection range of $360°$. The angular projection range utilized must correspond to at least the sum of $180°$ and the aperture angle of the scan beam fan. The possibility of segmental reconstruction is used to achieve especially short scanning times, improve the temporal resolution for CT scan series and occasionally for suppressing motion-induced → artifacts after scanning, if the movement producing the artifact occurs in only a limited angular projection region.

Semiconductor detector
Solid state → detector consisting of a semiconducting material which produces an electrical signal (current or voltage) through interaction with X-radiation. Frequently used synonymously with the term solid state → detector.

Sensitivity
Ratio of change in output signal to change in input signal, such as for an amplifier or a → detector.

167

Sensitivity, local
Ratio of change in output signal to change in input signal in a particular region of detector elements.

Sensitivity profile
Signal in the CT image corresponding to an object extending only very little in the direction of the → system axis (in the ideal case, infinitesimally), normalized to the maximum signal value, as a function of the object position along a line parallel to the → system axis. The sensitivity profile can vary with the distance of this line from the system axis.

Shaping filter
Beam filter for which the thickness varies within the beam to be filtered. Shaping filters are employed in CT systems in order to reduce signal level differences in the object slice scanned resulting from differences in object thickness (such as between the center and edge of a patient's body). Total object thickness compensation is physically impossible, due to the natural variations of the objects scanned and the deviations from circular geometry which these objects show. The use of a shaping filter makes it necessary to perform an individual → beam hardening correction for each scanning channel. See also → object thickness compensator.

Sigma value
Commonly used term for → standard deviation.

Signal-to-noise ratio
Quotient of the signal level to the → standard deviation of the noise level superimposed onto the signal.

Skin dose
Dose value produced at the surface of the patient's body.

Slice plane
Reference plane, oriented perpendicular to the → system axis and centered within the objects slice to be imaged.

Slice thickness
→ FWHM of the → sensitivity profile.

Software
General term for all computer programs.

Spatial frequency
Reciprocal of the periodic length for a spatially periodic structure.

Standard deviation
The standard deviation of a quantity which is subject to random processes and has been measured in a number of samples is the square root of the quotient found from the sum of the squares of the individual deviations from the average value to one less than the number of sample values.

Designating
n the number of sample values,
x_i the individual scan values,
$\bar{x}$ the average scan value and
σ the standard deviation,
then

$$\sigma = \sqrt{\frac{\sum_{i=1}^{n}(x_i - \bar{x})^2}{n-1}}$$

Stationary anode (X-ray) tube
X-ray tube with anode rigidly fixed to tube body. In general, the anode in such a tube is cooled by a fluid. Due to the good heat dissipation which results, these tubes are characterized by a relatively high long-term power rating. On the other hand, the peak loading is considerably less than that for → rotating anode (X-ray) tubes.

Storage, peripheral
→ Data storage addressed as an auxiliary device, as opposed to the working → storage of the → central processing unit. Data are stored there which are not frequently required for computational steps. Typical peripheral storage devices are magnetic tape floppy disc and LASER disc.

Storage, working
→ Data storage integrated into a computer, which the → central processing unit and arithmetic unit can address at any time and in which the program currently

running is stored. Because of the very short access times required, working storage consists almost exclusively of semiconductor memory, which has relegated the core memory of earlier times to almost total obsolescence.

Surface dose
See → skin dose.

System axis
Axis of rotation for the scanning system (X-ray tube with detector) of a CT system).

System geometry
See → imaging geometry.

System software
Term for all computer programs belonging to a CT scanning system.

Test program
Computer program for identification and localization of faulty computer hardware and software performance.

Text monitor
TV device for display of program texts and CT system operating dialog. See also → image monitor.

Time sharing
Simultaneous use of computational capacity of a computer by several programs or users, such that the → operating system regulates user or program access to the → central processing unit according to predefined priority system. See also → foreground-background operation.

Topogram
Designation for → digital survey scan performed with the SOMATOM.

Transfer function
See → modulation transfer function.

Translation-rotation operation
Operation of a → hybrid scanner as a → translation-rotation scanner.

Translation-rotation scanner
CT scanner for which the scanning system, consisting of X-ray tube and → detector arrangement, executes linear scanning movements parallel to the → slice plane in order to determine the → attenuation profiles and, following each translational movement, rotates about the → system axis to the next projection direction.

USRLIB
SOMATOM → program library allowing the system user to address the display unit, in particular the → image display memory, from user-formulated → FORTRAN IV programs running on the CT system. This greatly simplifies constructing the user's own evaluation programs.

Vignetting
Gradual, systematic changing of a CT value in the image of a homogeneous object toward the outer edge. The cause is frequently an inadequate → beam hardening correction.

Water cooling
Cooling system, such as for X-ray tubes, using water as the heat transfer medium. For a given flow volume, water cooling is considerably more efficient than → oil cooling, owing to its higher heat capacity. Due to problems of electrical insulation, however, water can only be used to cool an → anode held at ground potential. For some → stationary anode tubes, this is the case, so that CT scanners with these X-ray tubes employ water cooling. In all other cases, it is necessary to use oil cooling, which may entail cooling the oil itself by means of water.

Water phantom
See → phantom, water.

Winchester technology
Magnetic disc storage technology characterized by extremely high recording density. The recording density is the result of very high demands on mechanical precision and absence of dust in the system.

Window display
Selected display of a partial region from the CT values of a computed tomogram,

with full intensity range of the → image monitor. Image matrix elements with CT values lying outside of the selected range ("window") are displayed as black or white (color display functions analogously).

X-ray quantum
For X-radiation of given wavelength or frequency, lowest amount of energy which can interact with matter. This amount is the product of Planck's constant and the frequency of the X-radiation.

X-ray tube, effective optical focal spot
See → focal spot, effective optical, of an X-ray tube.

X-ray tube, electronic focal spot
See → focal spot, electronic, of an X-ray tube.

X-ray tube focal spot
See → focal spot of an X-ray tube.

X-ray tube focus
See → focus of an X-ray tube.

X-ray tube, optical focal spot
See → focal spot, optical, of an X-ray tube.

X-ray tube power rating
Permissible amount of electrical energy converted in an X-ray tube per unit time.

For practical operation, the → X-ray tube peak power rating and long-term power rating are of particular importance. The first determines the dose possible for a given scanning time or, equivalently, the scanning time required to reach a given dose level. The second determines how many scans are possible on the average per unit time for a given rate of energy conversion. The greatest number of scans possible in a fast series for a given rate of energy conversion is determined, on the other hand, by the heat storage capacity of the X-ray tube. See also → anode loading capacity.

X-ray tube peak power rating
See → X-ray tube pulse power rating.

X-ray tube pulse power rating
Permissible amount of electrical energy converted in an X-ray tube per unit time when the tube is switched on for a short time. See also → anode loading capacity and → X-ray tube power rating.

Zeroing
See → offset adjustment.

Zoom factor
Ratio of object diameter seen by scanning system to diameter of entire object region in the image. The object region displayed is determined by the zoom factor and the → reconstruction center.

Subject index

Absorption capability of detector 32
Acceptance 103
Add-on capacity 140
Air calibration 49
Algorithm 33
Algorithm and resolution 21
Aliasing 59
Aneurysm 104
Angio CT 103
Angle of irradiation 48
Angular velocity of X-ray tube 54
Anode heat loading capacity 108
Anode, high-performance 143
Anode loading 48
Anode loading capacity 48
Anode load monitoring 48
Anode roughening 48
Anti-scatter collimation 57, 63
Applicable dose level 49
Area noise 33
Archiving 84
Arithmetic unit 71
Array 71
Arrey processor 71, 114
Arteriovenous deformation 104
Artifact 45
Artifact behavior 58
Artifact correction 78
Aspects of routine applications 85
Attenuation capacity 18, 41
Attenuation properties 26
Attenuation value 134
Auto CT 103, 107, 109
Automatic zeroing 66

Back projection 72
Bar test 16, 17
Basic CT scanner types 51
Beam filtration 32
Beam hardening correction 18
   as a compromise 44, 45
Beam hardening effect 43
Beam hardening errors 18
Beam hardening problems 103

Beam intensity 43
Beam quality 38, 41, 43, 64
Beam width 18, 19
Biopsy 110
   and stereotaxis 110
Blood vessel pulsation 50
Blurring 50
Bolus 107
Bolus injection 109
Bore hole test 13
BSP 11 fast image processor 71, 77
Bus system 71

Cardio CT 50, 60, 103, 109
Center of reconstruction 26
Central processing unit 71
Central scan field 46
Chamber length of detector 61
Chamber voltage of detector 62
Chronogram 121
Cine-fluorography 137
Coarse-grained noise 35
Collimation of scattered radiation 57, 63
Collimator 29
Compound anode, high-performance 143
Compressed data storage 83
Computational effort 66
Computed radiogram 59
Computed radiography 58
Computer-supported
   therapy planning 114
Continuous beam operation 65
Contrast-detail diagram 37
   comparison for different CT systems 40
Contrast level discrimination
   capability 38, 40
Contrast medium dynamics 109
Control of scanner operation 33
Convolution 10, 50, 72
Cool-down rate 137
Cooperation of patient 49
Copper filter 44
Correlation 33
Cost-effectiveness analysis 130

171

Cost-effectiveness of CT systems 129
CT data correction 43
CT dose index (CTDI) 32
CT hardware 127
CT problems and goals 114
CT scanning system, general requirements for operation 85
CT scanner testing 33
CT software 77, 138, 141, 142
CT value falsification 57
Current-voltage converter 69

Data acquisition 71
Data acquisition channel 49
   sensitivity 49
Data acquisition rate 66, 71
Data field 71
Data processing 69
Data transfer 71
Density determination 41, 46
Density resolution capability 37
Detector 29
   absorption capability 32
   arrangement 54
   chamber voltage 62
   characteristics 62
   construction 61
   efficiency 108
   geometry 54
   grid 19
   inactive layer 63
   linear operating region 69
   local sensitivity 29
   number comprising array 53, 54
   pulse decay time 62
   system 107
   types 61
Dialog monitor 75
Dialog, operational 95
Digital image 97
Digital radiography 118
Digital survey scan 11
Direct measurement 17
Diskette drive 76
DMC 75, 77
Doping 62
Dose level 26
Dose profile 31
Dose utilization 19
Double window 79
DSC 76, 77

Dual-energy scanning method 45, 66, 90, 124
Dynamic computed tomography 97, 103

ECG-gated scan 103, 107
ECG-synchronized reconstruction 50
Edge-enhancing algorithm 21, 23
Edge response function 16, 17
Ejection fraction 115
Electronics components 32
Electronics noise 33
EMI scanner 10
Entrance window 63
Evaluation of CT cardiac images 115
Evaluation software 109
Examination procedure, flexibility 89

Fan-beam scanner 46, 50, 63
Filtration of beam 32
Fine-grained noise 13, 35
Fixed anode X-ray tube 53
Fluorescent material 62
Focal spot 18, 19, 29
   size 56
Followup studies 48
Foreground-background operation 77
FORTRAN IV 77
FWHM of sensitivity profile 26

Gantry 86
   aperture 88, 103
Gas detector 61, 62, 63, 138
Generation of X-ray beam 64
Groedel technique 57

Heater current 48
Heat loading capacity of anode 108
High contrast sensitivity 107
High dose level technique 98
High-performance compound anode 143
High-resolution algorithm 33
High-resolution CT 98
High-resolution detector 21
High-resolution modes 78
High-voltage generator, tuned 137
Homogeneity 41
   and beam hardening correction 41
   and quantitative diagnosis 43
   and shaped filter 43
Homogeneous water phantom 40
Host computer 71, 76, 77, 138

Hounsfield unit 134
Hybrid scanner 53

Image contrast, normalized 18
Image display memory 73
Image documentation and archiving 95
Image falsification due to movement
 of patient 75
Image monitor 75
Image postprocessing 115
Image quality 13
Image quality, optimized 98
Image rate 108
Image reconstruction 71
 algorithm 18
 and evaluation 90
 memory 72
Image sharpness 134
Inactive layer of detector 63
Indicator lights 88
Inert gas detector 61, 62, 63, 138
 saturation effect in 43
Inherent filtration 44, 48
Inhomogeneities caused by objects outside
 of the scan field 46
Input amplifier 69
Input device 138
Integrator stage 69
Interpretation of technical data 13

Lesion 102
Limiting diameter 16
Limiting frequency 16
Limiting spatial resolution 38
Linear operating region of detector 69
Local sensitivity of detector 29
Longitudinal dose product 32
Long-term archiving 97
Long-term power rating 52

Magnetic disc drive 76
Magnetic tape unit 76
Main console (DMC) 75
Maintenance 147
Matrix and resolution 23
Medical research 114
Medium-frequency generator 48
Metal-graphite alloy anode 66
Minicomputer 71, 112
Minimum contrast level 40
Mode of X-ray tube operation 65

Modular construction 141
Modulation transfer function (MTF)
 13, 16, 17, 18, 55
Monitor 97
Monitoring of anode loading 48
Monoenergetic CT scan 124
Morphology 41, 103
Movement of patient and image
 falsification 66
MTF calculation 16, 17
Multiformat magazine camera 83
Multiplexing 69
Multispot M 83

Needle puncture biopsy 110
Neighboring effect 18
Noise and noise structure 32
Noise from pixels 32
Noise level value 32
Noise structure and appearance
 of image 35
Noise structure and object form 35
Normalized image contrast 18
Number of detectors comprising
 array 53, 54
Nutation 56
Nyquist theorem 59

Offset adjustment 49
Oil cooling 52
Operating system 77, 138
 magnetic disc 79
Operational mode of X-ray tube 65
Operation of CT scanning system,
 general requirements 85
Optical memory 97
Optimized image quality 98
Optimized sensitivity profile 98

PACS 97
Parenchymal organ 104
Partial volume artifact 27
Partial volume effect 134
Patient cooperation 49
Patient dose efficiency 32
Patient dose level 26
Patient positioning 46, 86
PDP11 assembler 77
Peripheral data storage 71
Phantom 17, 29, 38, 40, 41
Photodiode 138

Pile-up factor 31
Pipeline principle 72
Pixel 23, 33
Pixel noise 33
Point of measurement 18
Point spread function 16, 17
Printer 116
Problems and goals of CT 114
Program 141
Prospective gating 109
Pulsed operation 66
Purchase costs 130

Quality control program 127
Quality standard 142, 145
Quality testing 145
Quantitative computed tomography 102
Quantitative density determination 46
Quantum 43, 64
Quantum efficiency 108
Quantum noise 32
Quarter detector offset 59

Radiation loss 64
Radiation therapy planning 112
Radioactive seed 110
Raw data correction 43
Reconstructions along curves 80
Rectangular modulation 16, 18
Reliability of scanner 134
Repairs 147
Reproducibility 48, 143
Resistor pen 79
Ring-shaped artifact 49
ROI 80
Rotating anode X-ray tube 53
Rotating detector 54
Rotating scanner 53
Routine applications 85
Routine examination 45

Safety checkout 147
Sampling characteristics 59
Sampling theorem 59
Sampling pulse frequency of detector 54
Saturation effect in inert gas detector 43
Scan 89
Scan field 46
Scanner operation control 33
Scanner reliability 134
Scanning electronics 69, 107

Scanning frequency 49, 89, 108
Scanning geometry and resolution 18
Scanning hardware 69
Scanning parameter selection 89
Scanning time 48
Scanning voltage 64
Scattered radiation collimation 57, 63
Scintillation crystal 63
Scintillation detector 63
Secondary slice 80
Segmental reconstruction 49
Semi-automatic examination sequence 141
Semiconductor detector 61
Sensitivity profile 26
Serio CT 108
Sequential CT 103
Shaping filter 37, 43, 46
Sharpness of image 35, 134
Signal falsification 66
Signal-to-noise ratio 66
Simultaneous rotation of X-ray tube and
   detector array 11
Skin dose 41
Slice summation method 116
Soft structures of body 23
Software 77, 100, 141, 142
Software-controlled magazine camera 97
Spatial frequency 18
Spatial resolution 13
Special applications 60, 97
Split image 108
Standard detector array 21
Stationary anode X-ray tube 53
Stationary detector ring 19, 54
Stereotactic frame 110
Stereotactic operating procedure 110
Subprogram library 80, 116, 121, 122, 127
Surface dose 31
Surface-length method 116
System concept 51, 139, 140
System servicing 146
System software 48

Temporal resolution 49
Therapy planning,
   computer-supported 114
Time sharing 77
Three-dimensional radiation
   therapy planning 114
Topogram 80, 97
   as diagnostic aid 118

Transit time method   123
Translation-rotation scanner   51, 52
Tuned high-voltage generator   137

Uncompressed data storage   83
USRLIB   80, 116, 121, 122, 127
Utilization of dose   19

Vignetting   43, 46, 47

Water cooling   52
Water phantom   17, 40
   homogeneous   40
Whole-body CT scanner   11, 144
Winchester technology   76
Window, double   79
Window setting   73
Wire phantom   17

X-radiation   32
X-ray beam generation   64
X-ray quantum   43, 64
X-ray signal   49
X-ray tube   43
   and detectory array   11
   simultaneous rotation
   of angular velocity   54
   current   48
   current regulator   48
   operational mode   65
   output   19
   voltage   48

Zeroing, automatic   66
Zoom factor   26, 78